Natacha Lescaille Elias

Diagnostic Ultrasound Topics

Natacha Lescaille Elias

Diagnostic Ultrasound Topics

for Imaging Technologists

ScienciaScripts

Imprint

Any brand names and product names mentioned in this book are subject to trademark, brand or patent protection and are trademarks or registered trademarks of their respective holders. The use of brand names, product names, common names, trade names, product descriptions etc. even without a particular marking in this work is in no way to be construed to mean that such names may be regarded as unrestricted in respect of trademark and brand protection legislation and could thus be used by anyone.

Cover image: www.ingimage.com

This book is a translation from the original published under ISBN 978-3-8417-5720-3.

Publisher:
Sciencia Scripts
is a trademark of
Dodo Books Indian Ocean Ltd. and OmniScriptum S.R.L publishing group

120 High Road, East Finchley, London, N2 9ED, United Kingdom
Str. Armeneasca 28/1, office 1, Chisinau MD-2012, Republic of Moldova, Europe
Printed at: see last page
ISBN: 978-620-5-88878-0

Contents

Main Authors

Prof. Natacha Lescaille EKas: Graduate in Health Technology. Specialist in Imaging. Doctor in Medical Education Science. Master of Science in Education. National methodologist of the careers in the area of Health Technologies of the Ministry of Public Health. President of the National Commission of the Degree Course in Medical Imaging and Radiography. Associate Researcher. Full Professor.

Prof. Armando Gonzalez Perez: Graduate in Health Technology. Specialist in Imaging. Master in Imaging Technology. Head of the Department of Health Technology. Member of the National Commission of the Degree in Medical Imaging and Radiography. Faculty of Medical Sciences General Calixto Garrta. Assistant Professor.

Prof. Suleyka Cabello Dasa: Graduate in Health Technology. Specialist in Imaging. Master in Imaging Technology. Member of the National Commission of the Degree in Medical Imaging and Radiography. Faculty of Health Technology. Assistant Professor.

Prof. Beatriz Borrero Sanchez: Graduate in Health Technology. Specialist in Imaging. Master in Imaging Technology. Faculty of Health Technology. Instructor Professor.

<u>**Contributors:**</u>

Prof. Carlos Manuel Breijo Garcia: Bachelor in Education. Speciality Biology. Main Professor of Imaging Profile. Member of the National Commission of the Degree in Medical Imaging and Radiography. Faculty of Health Technology. Assistant Professor.

Prof. Rolando Wilson Calderin: Bachelor of Education. Speciality Biology. Head of the Department of Medical Imaging and Radiography. Member of the National Commission of the Degree in Medical Imaging and Radiography. Faculty of Health Technology. Assistant Professor.

Prof. Aymara Enrique Zambrana: Graduate in Health Technology. Specialist in Imaging. Master in Diagnostic Means. Member of the National Commission of the Degree in Medical Imaging and Radiography. Faculty of Health Technology. Assistant Professor.

Prof. Ana Milagro Ponce Rojas: Graduate in Health Technology. Specialist in Imaging. Faculty of Health Technology. Assistant Professor.

Chapter #1 Physics of Ultrasound.

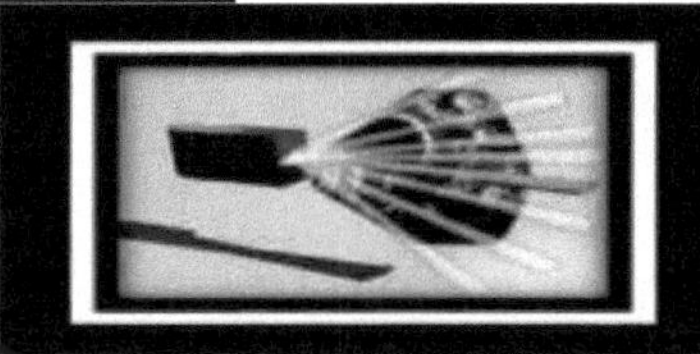

- ✓ Sound wave.
- ✓ Historical review.
- ✓ Transducers
- ✓ Physical events of the US in its interaction with tissues
- ✓ Working techniques. Modes
- ✓ Artefacts.

Chapter #2 Ultrasound Upper Hemiabdomen
Liver:

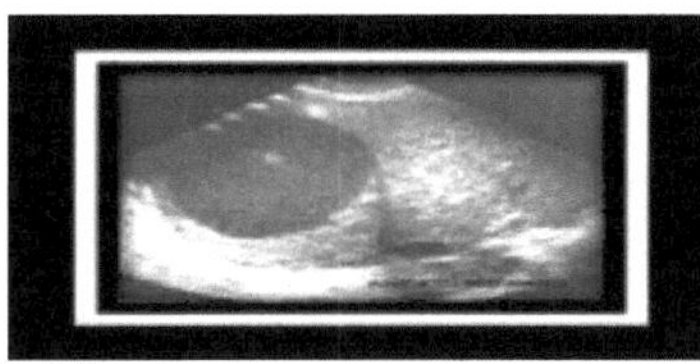

- ✓ Indications of the US of ^gado.
- ✓ Preparation and Technique.
- ✓ Normal liver appearance
- ✓ Size and shape of the liver.
- ✓ Pathological alterations.
- ✓ Diffuse hepatomegaly with homogeneous pattern.
- ✓ Diffuse inhomogeneous hepatomegaly.
- ✓ Small and retracted liver.
- ✓ Cystic lesion, normal or enlarged liver.
- ✓ Hepatic trauma.
- ✓ Differential diagnosis of a liver mass. Single solid mass. Abscess.

Bladder and Bile Ducts.

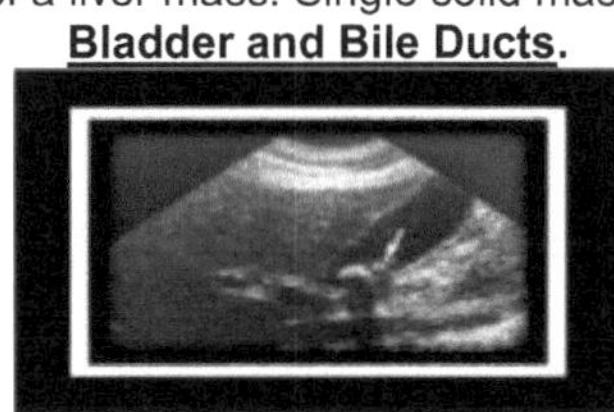

- ✓ Indications for Ultrasound of the Bladder and Biliary Tract.
- ✓ Anatom^a of the Vesfcula.
- ✓ Normal anatomy of the bile ducts.
- ✓ Normal gall bladder.
- ✓ Patient preparation.
- ✓ Ultrasound technique of the gallbladder and bile ducts.
- ✓ Normal variants of the vesicle.
- ✓ Pre- and post-pandral vesfcula.
- ✓ Pathological alterations I. (Non-visualisation of the Vesphcula).
- ✓ Pathological alterations II (distended bladder).

✓ Pathological alterations III (Presence of intravesicular echoes).
✓ Pathological alterations V. (Thickening of the vesicular wall).
✓ Pathological alterations (small vesicle).
✓ Bile duct dilatation.
✓ Obstructive Icterus.

Ultrasound of the spleen.

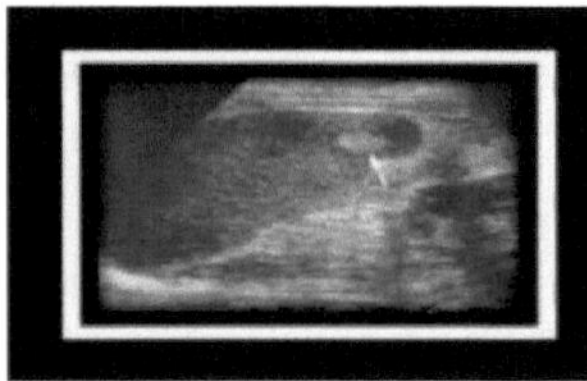

✓ Indications for US of the spleen.
✓ Preparation and Technique.
✓ Normal ultrasonographic anatomy of the spleen.
✓ Pathological alterations of the spleen.
✓ Diffuse splenomegaly.
✓ Well-defined cystic lesions.
✓ Ill-defined cystic lesion, abscesses.
✓ Intrasplenic mass.
✓ Febrile syndrome.
✓ Closed abdominal trauma.
✓ Portal hypertension.
✓ Tumours.
✓ Metastasis.
✓ Splenic infarcts.
✓ Trauma.

Ultrasound of the Pancreas

✓ Indications for US of the Pancreas.
✓ Preparation and Technique.
✓ Normal ultrasonographic appearance of the pancreas.
✓ Normal pancreas.
✓ Normal variants of the pancreas.
✓ Pathological alterations of the pancreas I. (Small pancreas).
✓ Pathological alterations of the pancreas II (diffuse enlargement of the pancreas).
✓ Direct signs of pancreatitis.
✓ Indirect signs of pancreatitis.
✓ Pancreatic abscess.
✓ Pathological alterations of the pancreas III (localised non-cystic enlargement).
✓ Pancreatic lymphoma.
✓ Pancreatic metastases.
✓ Pathological alterations of the pancreas IV (predominantly cystic localised enlargement).
✓ Pathological alterations of the pancreas V. (Pancreatic calcifications).

✓ Pathological alterations of the pancreas VI (pancreatic duct dilatation).

Renal Ultrasound.

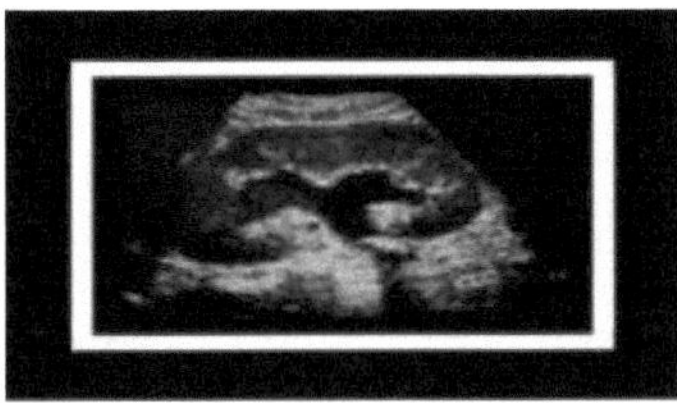

✓ Indications for renoureteral US.
✓ Preparation and Technique.
✓ Renal malformations.
✓ Pathological alterations of the kidney (renal absence).
✓ Renal pathologies.
✓ Obstruction of the excretory system.
✓ Infectious processes.
✓ Benign renal expansive processes.
✓ Malignant renal expansive processes.

Ultrasound of the adrenal gland

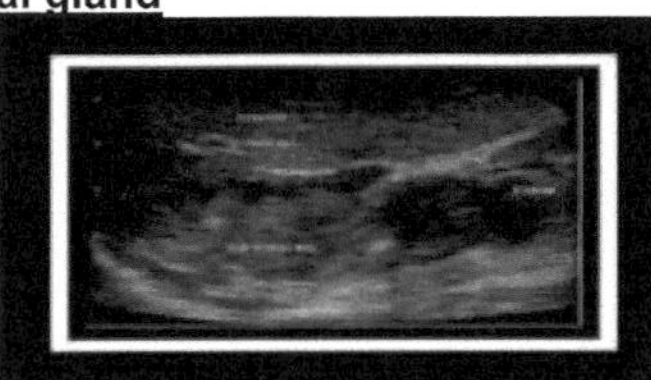

✓ Indications
✓ Preparation and Technique.
✓ Pathological alterations of GSRs.

Chapter #3 Ultrasound of the Lower Hemiabdomen

Bladder.

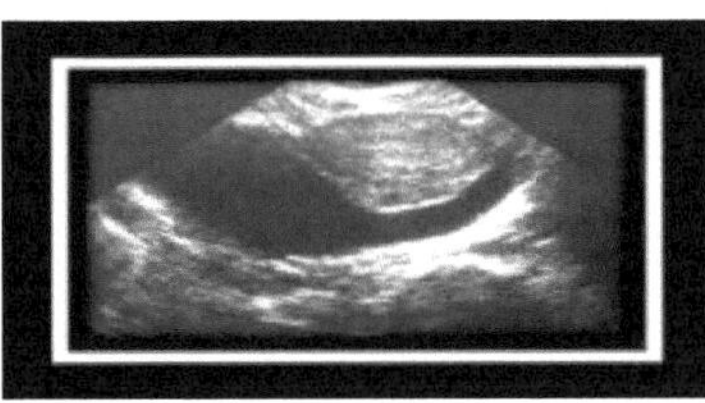

✓ Indications for US of the bladder.
✓ Approach routes for the US study of the bladder.
✓ Preparation and Technique.
✓ Functional study of the bladder.
✓ Repletion and post micturition examination.
✓ Normal anatomy of the bladder.
✓ Pathological alterations of the bladder.
✓ Generalised wall thickening.
✓ Localised wall thickening.
✓ Intravesical masses.
✓ Megavejiga.
✓ Small bladder.

✓ Pathological alterations of neighbouring organs.
✓ Traumatic bladder injuries.

<u>Prostate</u>

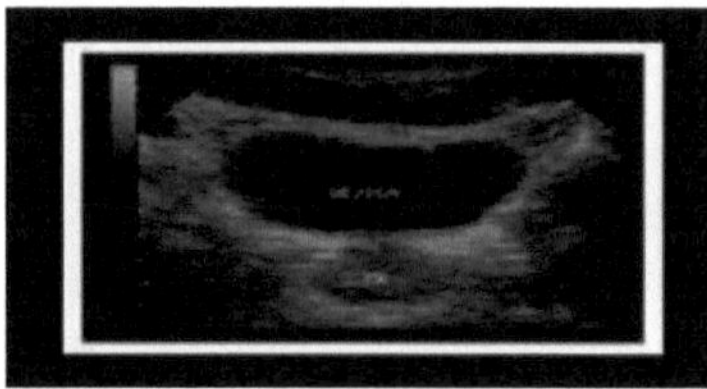

✓ Indications for prostate US.
✓ Approach routes for the US study of the prostate.
✓ Suprapubic abdominal route.
✓ Anatomy of the prostate.
✓ Ultrasonographic appearance of the prostate.
✓ Pathological alterations of the prostate (Prostatitis).

Seminal Vesfuculae.

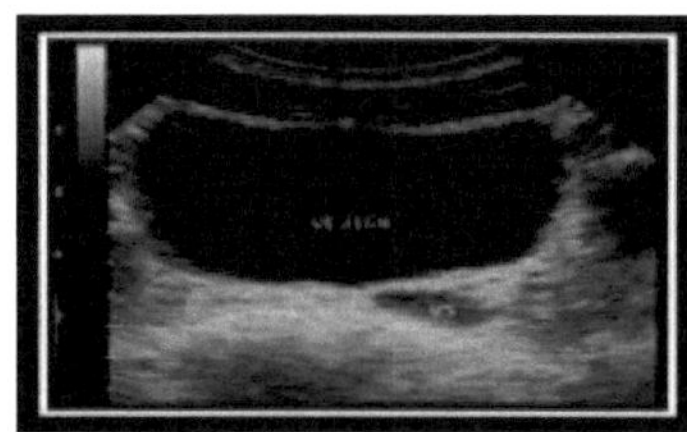

✓ Indications for seminal vesicle US.
✓ Ultrasonographic examination technique and anatomy.
✓ Most frequent pathological alterations.

Chapter #4 Ultrasound of the Peritoneal Cavity and GIT.

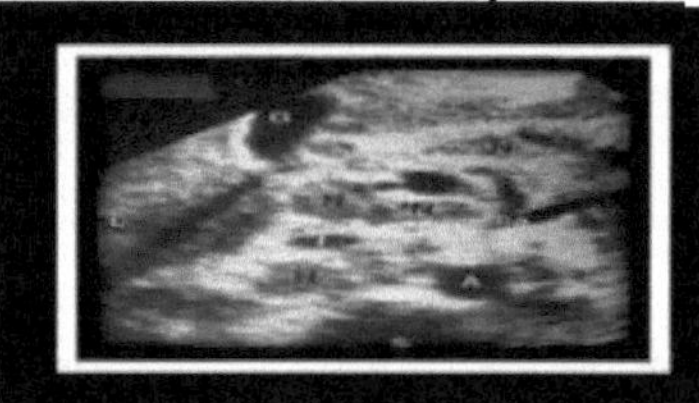

✓ Indications for US of the peritoneal cavity and GIT.
✓ Preparation and Technique.
✓ Normal anatomy of the GIT.
✓ Pathological alterations of the PC and TGI (hypertrophic pyloric stenosis).
✓ Appendicitis.
✓ Invagination.
✓ Parasitosis.
✓ Ascites.
✓ Intestinal masses.
✓ Extraintestinal masses.
✓ Complex masses.
✓ Haematomas.
✓ Masses full of Kquido.

✓ AIDS infection.

Chapter #5 Gynaecological and Obstetric Ultrasound.
Gynaecologist

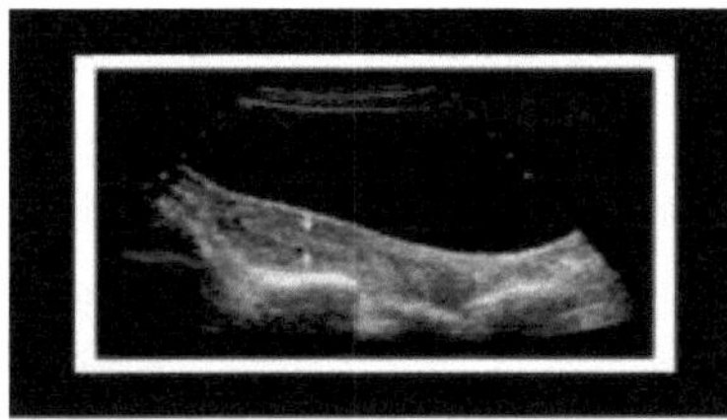

✓ Indications for gynaecological US.
✓ Preparation and Technique.
✓ Normal US anatomy of the gynaecological system
✓ Physiological variations of the endometrium. Normal endometrial thickness.
✓ Pathological alterations of the uterus (developmental abnormalities).
✓ Lesions inside the vagina.
✓ Cystic structures in the cervix.
✓ Enlargement and pathological alterations of the uterus.
✓ Fibromas.
✓ Malignant tumours.
✓ Increased endometrial thickness.
✓ Ovarian cycle.
✓ Pathological alterations of the ovary.
✓ Cysts. Simple adnexal cysts.
✓ Complex adnexal mass.
✓ Ovarian tumours.

Obstetrics and foetal biometry.

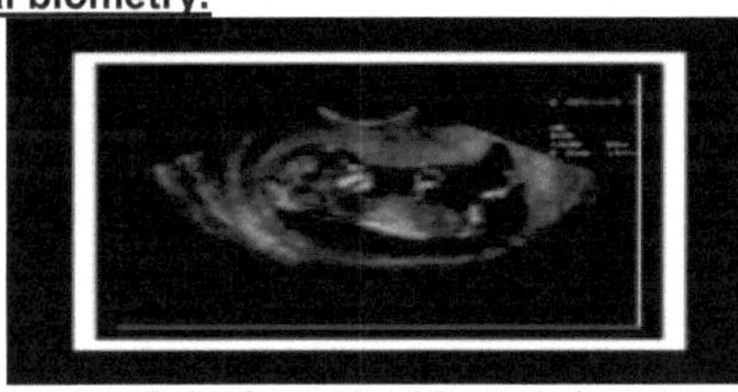

✓ Indications for obstetric US (before 18 - 22 weeks).
✓ Importance of obstetric US (18 - 22 weeks).
✓ Importance of obstetric US (32 - 36 weeks).
✓ Early pregnancy.
✓ IUD.
✓ Ectopic pregnancy.
✓ Embryo.
✓ Yolk sac and yolk sac.
✓ Multiple pregnancy.
✓ First trimester disturbances.
✓ Enlarged uterus.
✓ Obstetric study algorithm.
✓ Obstetric examination. Fetal biometry
✓ Measurement of DBP.
✓ Fronto-occipital diameter measurement.

✓ Cephalic Hdice.
✓ Head circumference index.
✓ Abdominal circumference.
✓ Measurement of long bones.
✓ Recognition of CIUR.
✓ Determination of gestational age.

Chapter #6 Ultrasound of small parts
Scrotum and Testis.

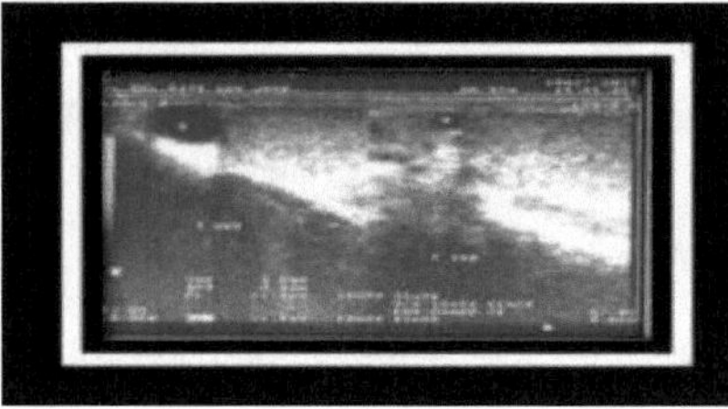

✓ Indications for US of the scrotum and testicles.
✓ Preparation and Technique.
✓ Testicular anatomy.
✓ Pathological alterations.
✓ Hernia.
✓ Torsion of the testicular appendix.
✓ Epididymitis.
✓ Orchitis.
✓ Cyst of the epididymis or testis.
✓ Hydrocele. Varicocele.
✓ Spermatocele.
✓ Testicular trauma.
✓ Atrophy.
✓ Calcifications.
✓ Abscesses.
✓ Tumours.
✓ Germ cell tumours:
✓ Tumours of the sexual cords and gonadal stroma.
✓ Non-specialised testicular stromal tumours.
✓ Metastatic or secondary tumours.
✓ Pathological alterations (pseudotumours).
✓ Pathological alterations (malignant tumours).
✓ Testicular pathological alterations (metastasis).

Thyroid Gland

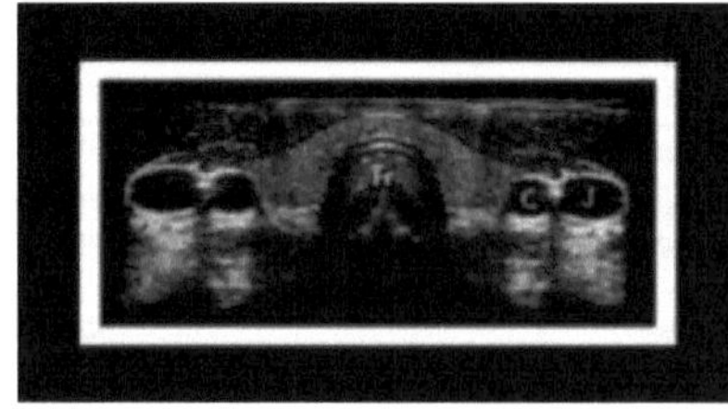

✓ Indications for thyroid US.
✓ Preparation and technique.

- ✓ Normal anatomy of the neck.
- ✓ Location and anatomy of the thyroid.
- ✓ Thyroid anomaKas.
- ✓ Increase in the volume of the neck.
- ✓ Pathological alterations of the thyroid (homogeneous diffuse enlargement).
- ✓ Causes of goitre. US image of goitre.
- ✓ Thyroiditis.
- ✓ Thyroid nodules.
- ✓ Pathological alterations of the thyroid (heterogeneous enlargement).
- ✓ Pathological alterations of the thyroid (localised cystic masses).
- ✓ Pathological alterations of the thyroid (localised mixed masses).
- ✓ Pathological alterations of the thyroid (malignant nodules).

Neck vessels (carotid and vertebral).

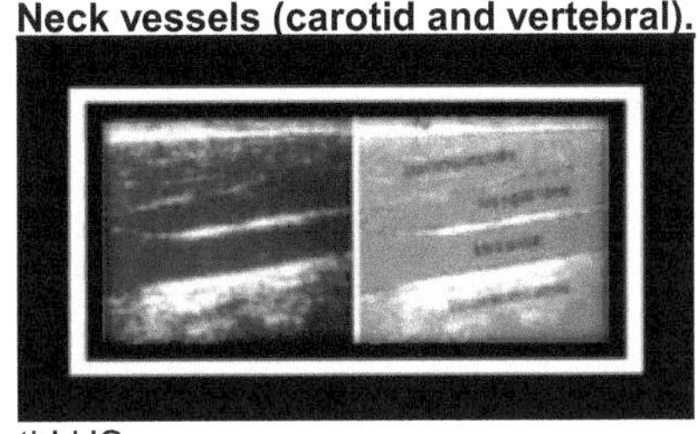

- ✓ Indications for carotid US.
- ✓ Preparation.
- ✓ Technique for the study of the vessels of the neck.
- ✓ Colour Doppler ultrasound of the vertebral artery.

<u>Mama</u>

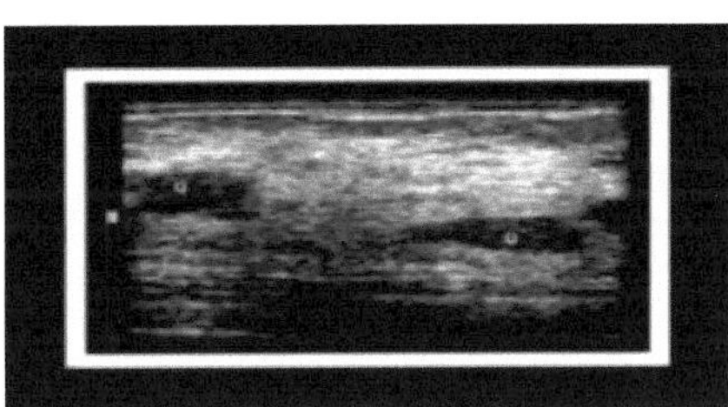

- ✓ Indications for breast US.
- ✓ Normal anatomy.
- ✓ Examination technique.
- ✓ Normal sonographic appearance of the breast.
- ✓ Pathological sonographic appearance of the breast.

Chapter #1
Physics of Ultrasound.
Historical review.

1914. 1st World War. French Government commissions physicist Langevin and SONAR is created.
1939. 2nd World War. SONAR reaches its maximum development.
1942. Dussik Bros. visualise brain ventricles using sound.
1950. The first US images are obtained.
1979. The US is introduced in Cuba.
Year 1880. The Curies discovered a property in quartz crystals which they called: PIEZOELECTRICITY. This property is also attributable to other materials such as Rochelle salt and lithium sulphate or can be artificially induced in certain ceramics...
Definition of wave, (from the physical point of view)
• It is the modification of a physical medium, product of an initial perturbation that propagates through it, in the form of periodic oscillations. It can be summarised as the propagation of a particle of any material body produced by a determined force or action, which causes the adjacent particle to vibrate in space and in this way propagates through the whole body. Shaft. An object in water.
Types of waves
• Electric wave: it is the one produced by current-carrying bodies.
• Electromagnetic wave: originates from a magnetic field.
• Mechanical wave: it needs a material body for its propagation, sound is not transmitted in a vacuum.
For the propagation of mechanical waves, physical bodies are considered to consist of particles connected by springs, which means that if the particle moves to the left, the spring on the right is stretched, if the displaced particle is released, it will be attracted to its initial position, but if it exceeds this initial position, it will move to the right because of the spring that connects it, If the displaced particle is released, it will be attracted to its initial position, but if it exceeds this initial position, it will move to the right because of the spring that connects it, until the spring effect stops, in this way the particle spreads to the left and to the right of its resting position.
This happens until the frictional force is greater than the spring effect, so that the vibration cycle of the particle is less than the previous one at each moment until it is zero, producing a small amount of energy used to overcome the frictional force, giving off some heat. All this happens because the connection between the particles is elastic, if it were rigid then all the particles would move at the same time and to the same side in perfect synchronisation, but because of the elastic connection there is a finite delay between the movement of one particle and that of its neighbour, giving rise to different types of mechanical waves.
Types of mechanical waves
• Longitudinal waves: the particles vibrate in the same direction as the wave.
• Transverse waves: Particle vibrations vibrate transverse or perpendicular to the wave motion.
• Surface waves: vibrations of particles occur at the surface of bodies.
The ones we are interested in are the longitudinal mechanical waves, which have their own characteristics.
Characteristic of a longitudinal mechanical wave.
• **Cycle: The** complete path of a wave or vibration.
• **Wavelength:** It is the distance that exists between the peaks of maximum pressure located consecutively. It is the most important element as it determines the

resolution capacity of a sound beam.
- **Period (P):** The time taken to complete a cycle is measured in seconds.
- **Frequency (F):** Number of cycles that pass through a point in one second. Its unit is one cycle/sec, called Hertz (Hz). The frequency is the inverse of the period: F=1/P. It is the number of oscillations (vibration or cycle) of a particle per unit of time (second). Frequency is measured in Hertz (Hz). One Hertz is one oscillation (cycle) per second. As ultrasound is a high frequency wave, the basic measure used is the Megahertz (MHz), which is equal to one million Hz.
- **Amplitude (A):** The maximum distance of separation of a point of the cycle in relation to the equilibrium position. It is measured in units of length. Amplitude is related to intensity. Thus, if we increase the intensity of a given wave, we increase its amplitude. During the transmission of waves, due to the effect of their interaction with the medium, the intensity of the wave decreases as a function of the distance travelled and, as a consequence, its amplitude decreases. The physical unit used to represent the amplitude of ultrasound is the belio, but in practice the decibel (dB), which is one tenth of a belio, is used.
- **Velocity:** The propagation velocity is the distance travelled by the wave divided by the time taken to travel that distance. The speed of ultrasound in a given tissue depends on the density and elasticity of the medium, which in turn vary with temperature. The relationship is direct, i.e. the higher the density of the medium, the higher the speed of ultrasound transmission. However, the speed depends on the temperature.
- **Intensity:** The energy that passes per second through a surface of unit area placed perpendicular to the direction of propagation of the movement. Intensity decreases with distance.

Sound waves are longitudinal mechanical waves and specifically they are the protagonists in Diagnostic Ultrasound.

<u>Classification of sound, according to human hearing ability.</u>
- Infrasound waves or infrasound.

(Inaudible waves, as they are not picked up by the human ear, have frequencies of less than 20 Hz).
- Sound waves or sound.

(comprised between the limits of hearing), because if they are picked up by the human ear, they present frequencies between 20 and 20,000 Hz or 20 KHz, since 1 KHz is equivalent to 1000 Hz and 1 MHz is equivalent to 1000 KHz.
- high tones (high frequencies)
- low tones (low frequencies)
- Ultrasonic waves or ultrasound.

(Inaudible waves, as they are not picked up by the human ear and have frequencies above 20,000Hz).

<u>Definition of US</u>
These are mechanical vibrations of matter that are transmitted in the form of pressure waves. Ultrasound propagates in the form of longitudinal waves; in this type of wave, the direction of propagation coincides with the direction of vibration. The wave is transmitted in the form of successive cycles of condensation and rarefaction of matter.

In order to propagate through a medium, the medium must have two properties: inertia and elasticity. Unlike audible waves, ultrasound cannot be transmitted through air, because the higher the frequency, the higher the density/support of the medium is required for transmission.

Ultrasound will have a very important characteristic that differentiates it from lower frequency sounds, namely directionality, i.e. the ultrasonic wave does not propagate in all directions but forms a small beam that can be "focused". Furthermore, in a similar way to what happens with a light wave, acoustic lenses can be applied which can modulate the ultrasonic beam. This allows us to focus our beam on the area to be explored, leaving out of focus those that are located in front or behind that point, that is to say, the same as with light waves, there is the concept of "depth of focus", which would apply to all the structures that are focused using a beam of certain characteristics.

This wave is used in ultrasound scanners. When the equipment is connected to the power supply, electrical energy enters and with the presence of transducers, which are nothing more than devices that convert one energy into another, in this case into sound energy. For the conversion of electrical energy into ultrasonic energy, special transducers are needed, which contain inside them materials with the property of piezoelectricity, such as quartz or tourmaline, as well as crystals obtained in the laboratory such as Rochelle or Seignette salt or ceramic mixtures such as barium titanate and lead zirconate.

Ultrasonic waves, unlike electromagnetic waves, need a material support for their propagation. However, this is produced without transporting matter **but** energy. As we have seen, the amplitude and intensity of the emitted wave decreases with distance, so the amplitude of the echo received by our instrument decreases. This is due to the interaction of the wave with the tissue, since during its propagation, the wave loses energy, limiting its penetration into the tissue. When this wave interacts with living tissue, a series of physical processes take place, which we will summarise below.

<u>Historical Processes</u>

•   <u>Acoustic impedance</u>: This is the capacity of a medium to transmit sound; it is the opposition offered by a medium to the passage of the acoustic wave, which will depend on the properties of that medium. We have seen that when an ultrasound beam passes through a medium, its speed depends on the density and elasticity of the medium. The acoustic impedance is the product of the density of the tissue and the velocity of the ultrasound beam passing through it; it reflects the elastic properties of the tissue and is the main characteristic of the tissue from an ultrasonic point of view.

•   <u>Interface</u>: A surface that separates two different media for the passage of sound.

•   <u>Reflection</u>: It is the fundamental process in the production of the echo (What is the echo), to point out that only the waves that fall perpendicular to the interfaces will arrive in the form of echo to the crystal, and that when they arrive a portion of the sound is reflected backwards and the rest continues its journey through the tissues, This process is important because if the echo does not arrive perpendicular to the interface, we will not have a reflected or transmitted beam, so we will not obtain any image, since the reflected beam is the image observed on the monitor and it must be reflected and transmitted. Axis: The air is the enemy of the USD because it has little acoustic impedance, that is to say, little capacity to transmit sound and almost nothing is transmitted. Bone also has a high acoustic impedance and the acoustic shadow is formed and everything is transmitted and we do not obtain a useful image. This is joined by another process, Refraction.

•   <u>Refraction</u>: it is nothing more than the beam transmitted in the previous process, conceptually, it is the change in direction that the sonic beam undergoes when it crosses an interface due to the change of the medium, in USD it is not diHcile since this change can be seen with the presence of calcification, of Kquido or of the bone.

•   <u>Dispersion</u>: occurs when the sound encounters an irregular surface and the particles are very small compared to the wavelength of the sound. In other words, it is the negative element in the formation of the image, it is the reflection of the beam in several directions due to the irregularity of several interfaces. The higher the degree of scattering, the worse the image is defined. Fatty tissue is the enemy of the USD. Obese people have a high degree of scattering.

•   <u>Absorption</u>: energy dissipation occurs when the sound interacts with the tissue and is transformed into heat, this process is used in therapeutic ultrasound. Absorption is directly proportional to the frequency used.

•   <u>Attenuation:</u> it is the reduction of the intensity of the beam, since the sound propagates through the matter and decreases progressively, this process must be avoided since the characteristics of the structure are lost and for this something artificial is done which is the compensation of the gain in time. The first thing is to choose the transducer and the second thing is to compensate the gain (TGC). The emission of the echo must be by pulse, not conthuo and between pulse and pulse there is a time and it is where you have to identify what arrives first and what arrives later, the closest and the furthest. The later is more amplified, the less late is less distorted. The gain control is represented by levels: - near, -far, -slope, -delay. (Graphically) The operator moves the curve depending on what he wants, I raise the near and bring the far closer, or vice versa.

•   <u>Resolution</u>: is the smallest distance at which 2 points can be observed as separate, i.e. the separation power, the ability of the sonic beam to distinguish different structures in close proximity. In US we see two planes, axial resolution for the depth (structures on top of each other) and lateral resolution for the lateral plane (structures next to each other).

•   <u>Image formation</u>: this is the process in which all the above processes come together, from the production of the echo at each interface this is deformed, due to the piezoelectric property of the crystal, then goes through an amplification stage by passing through the cathode tube or observation screen. The screen is positively charged and coated with phosphor in such a way that the stream of electrons will stick to the screen and produce a flash of light, each a reflection at an interface. The image will be the electronic representation of the overall data at the interfaces returning to the crystal and observed on the screen.

The Transducer

•   This is the element that contains the piezoelectric crystal(s), i.e. the US emitting and echo receiving crystals.

<u>Transducer Classification</u>

These are classified according to their type:

- Sectoral
- Linear
- Convex

Based on their use:

- Abdominals
- Echocardiography
- Transcavity
- For PB

By their mode of operation:

- Mechanics
- Electronics

Based on their frequency:

- Multifrequency (3.5 mhz to 10 mhz)

<u>Advantages of Transducers.</u>

Sector transducer

•   Wide glass path for better resolution.

- Window small enough to allow sound to penetrate between intercostal spaces.
- Wide scan angle, best for echocardiographic, transrectal and transvaginal transducers.

Linear transducer.
- Wide contact plane ideal for the study of muscles and tendons as well as small structures such as thyroid, testis, peripheral lymph nodes and breasts.
- They are typically 7.5 MHz to 10 MHz.

Convex transducer.
- Large distance contact with just the right window size.
- Electronic focus for better resolution at depth.
- It may include options for 3D and 4D programmes.
- Ideal for abdominal, gynaecological and obstetrical studies.

The crystals may be distributed in the transducer in a so-called "linear array" (the crystals are excited sequentially) or a "sectorial array" (the crystals are excited out of phase and give a cone of information that fans out as it progresses in depth). The crystals can be designed in the thickness mode and in the radial mode.

Design of the crystals.
- Thickness mode: Mode of choice in the formation of the US for diagnostics and it is the thickness of the crystal that determines its vibrational frequency, also called resonance frequency.
- Radial mode: Vibrates in the form of diverging rays from its centre to the periphery.

Working techniques. Modes.
- Mode A
- Mode M
- Mode B
- TR mode
- Doppler mode
- 3D mode
- 4D Mode

Mode A
- Amplitude mode.
- The echoes are represented as positive deflections on a horizontal baseline, with the first deflection on the left of the oscilloscope screen corresponding to the beginning of the ultrasonic pulse, the remaining deflections representing the different interfaces through which the sound travels.
- Maximum application: Encephalograffa and Ophthalmology.

Mode M
- Motion Mode.
- It is a variation of Mode A, the echoes will be represented as luminous points instead of positive deflections, the luminosity depending on the amplitude of the echo, in this mode the position and the movement is collected, being able to collect its register in a strip of paper that advances at a determined speed.
- Maximum Application: Echocardiography.

Mode B.
- Gloss.
- Echoes represented as luminous dots as in Mode M, but instead of being oriented from left to right on the oscilloscope screen, they are oriented in the same direction as the transducer, which is connected to an arm and the arm is connected to a computer which picks up the position of the echo location. Mode B has a memory and records all echoes and retains them on the screen.
- Maximum application: Abdomen.

<u>TR mode.</u>
- Real Time Mode.
- It is an advanced variant of Mode B, to which motion is imparted, either by placing crystals that move faster than the human eye can perceive or by placing many crystals that send their impulses with a small time difference from each other.
- Maximum application: obstetrics.
<u>Doppler mode.</u>
- 1842. Christian Johan Doppler raises:
"The frequency with which a wave emission is perceived by an observer increases as he approaches the emitting source and decreases as he moves away from it, and this is given by the compressions and stretches that occur in it, given that the speed of displacement is constant.
- A special technique used to determine the movement of small particles such as red blood cells in the blood.
- Maximum application: Haemodynamics.
- Doppler variants:
- Contmuo Doppler
- Pulsed Doppler
- Duplex Doppler
- Colour Doppler
- Angio Power
<u>3D mode.</u>
- Three-dimensional mode.
- Programmes created and applied for the post-processing of two-dimensional images capable of converting p^xels into pixels based on three planes: height, width and depth. The 3D images are static.
- Maximum application: obstetrics.
4D mode.
- Four-dimensional mode
- Very fast automatic post-processing programme that reconstructs and shapes 2D images into 3D by incorporating the time-motion element as a fourth dimension.
- Maximum application: obstetrics (Multipurpose)
Market launch: Year 2002
Equipment: GE Voluson 730 Expert
Artefacts.
Artefacts in the different CT and MRI imaging techniques degrade the images and reduce their diagnostic value.
Ultrasound is also subject to artefacts, i.e. echoes that do not correspond to real interfaces of the structures studied, but unlike the other techniques, in ultrasound some of these artefacts can be useful in establishing differences or making a diagnosis.
- Classification of Artefacts.
- Good (acoustic shading, rear reinforcement)
- Bad (Refraction, reverberation, anisotropic reflectors)
These should be known and the circumstances in which they may be encountered.
Good Artifacts.
- Acoustic shadow.
It occurs at highly reflective interfaces where all the incident sound energy is reflected away leaving a very small amount of energy useful for imaging.
Result: a signal is emitted from behind the hyper-reflective object.
Acoustic Shadow
- Classic examples where we can find this artefact:

-the bones
-   the air
-   musculo-tendinous calcifications
-   vesicular, renal, bladder and gall bladder stones
-   calcified breast nodules
-   calcified fibroids
-   arterial calcifications
•   Subsequent reinforcement.

Posterior reinforcement is also referred to as comet tail artifact. It occurs between interfaces where the acoustic impedance has a large variability.

Result: characteristic bands of increased echogenicity behind the studied structure or object (foreign body). These bands cross the tissue borders.

Rear Reinforcement
•   Classic examples of where we can find this artefact:
-   Kquid-filled cavities like the bladder
-   Cysts (hepatic, renal, breast)
-   Foreign bodies in Soft Parts (metal or glass)

Bad Artifacts.
•   Refraction.

Detection of real structures in a false localisation and occurs between tissue interfaces that transmit sound at very different speeds, the beam is bent between these interfaces in proportion to the differences in the speed of sound transmission.

Example: Interfaces between fat (1 450 m/s) and muscle (1 585 m/s)
•   Reverberation.

Phantom echoes occurring at highly reflective interfaces.

Example: Diaphragm, bladder full of urine, etc.

This effect is very harmful as it can lead to false diagnoses due to suspicion of non-existent lesions.
•   Anisotropic reflectors.

These are structures that exhibit different properties depending on the direction of the sound beam.

Examples: muscles and tendons have a marked anisotropy.

This effect can be eliminated or attenuated by making the sound beam as perpendicular as possible to the structure.

With increasing technology, the shape and size of transducers and of the ultrasound equipment itself have changed, making it easier to handle and to acquire numerical data on the amplitude of echoes in certain organs. These values are the product of a series of physical processes that are necessary to normalise in order to obtain quantitative data from an ultrasound image.

The Ultrasound technique is divided into:

Organisational stage:
1.   Calling the patient, rectifying the data and prior preparation.
2.   Explain to him/her the type of examination to be carried out for his/her cooperation.
3.   The equipment is programmed and the new patient data is entered.
4.   Previous studies are reviewed and the patient is questioned according to studies and clinical data.

Realisation of the Technique:
1.   Revision of the indication.
2.   Transducer selection.
3.   Use of the gel.
4.   Scanning sweep to verify readiness.

5.   Perform the different cuts (transverse, longitudinal or oblique).
6.   Search for normal and pathological landmarks.
7.   Mobilise the patient if necessary, instruct the patient on some manoeuvres to be performed during the study.
(Mastery of the equipment and the cuts made is required).
<u>The terminology used is varied:</u>
•   Echogenic: Term applied to tissues that produce brighter (Hyperechogenic or Hyperechoic.) or duller (Hypoechogenic or Hypoechoic) echoes than adjacent tissues, e.g. Hyperechoic. bones, peri renal fat, walls of the gall bladder and cirrhotic liver. Example of Hypo. lymph nodes, some tumours and kyphoid.
•   Mixed: It has characteristics of the two previous ones.
•   Isoechoic: Term used for a lesion whose characteristics are similar to the underlying tissue.
•   Anechoic, anechogenic, echogenic, echolucent: no echoes or except for echoes with posterior enhancement and blunt edges, fluid content, e.g. normal urine and bile.
•   Borders: mtidos suggestive of benignity, ill-defined and irregular, are highly suggestive of malignancy.
•   Side shadows: Two shadows supporting benignity.
•   A shadow: Other criteria supporting benignity should be sought.
•   Thin, complete halo very suggestive of benignity, e.g. in the case of thyroid nodules.
•   Thick, irregular haloes suggestive of rapid growth (malignancy)

Chapter 2

Ultrasound Upper Hemiabdomen

Ultrasound of the liver.
Indications for liver US.

1   Hepatomegaly.
2   Suspected liver abscess.
3   .- fctero.
4   Abdominal trauma.
5   Ascites.
6   Suspected tumour disease.
7   Pain in CSD.
8   Hydatid cyst screening.
9   As a guide for BAAF implementation.

Preparation and Technique.

Fasting patient.

A 3.5 to 5 MHz transducer is used and sagittal, transverse and subcostal slices are performed: intercostal slices are frequently performed, especially in cases where the patient is unable to take deep breaths (in case of emergency, the procedure is immediate). The patient can adopt an initial position in dorsal or supine decubitus, then in left lateral decubitus or left anteroposterior oblique.

Liver Anatomy

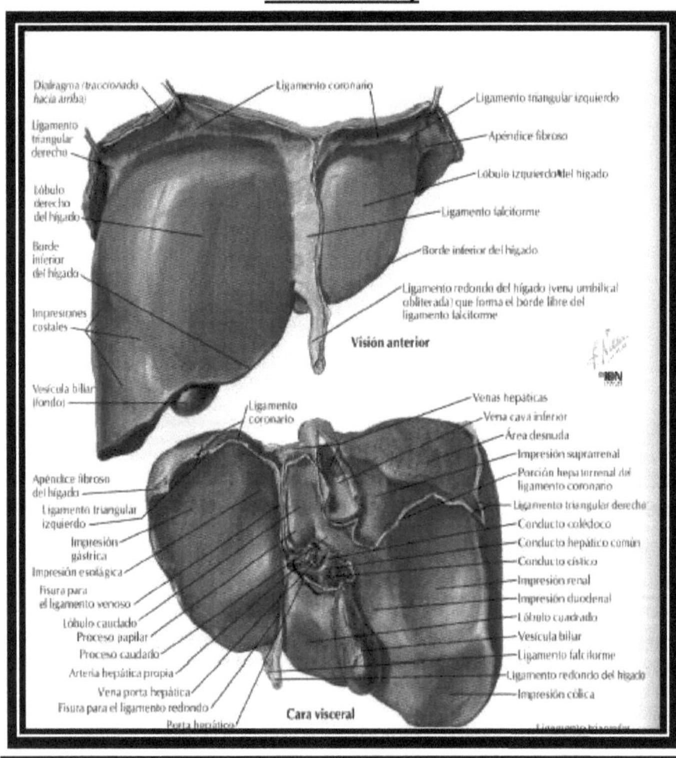

Anatomical variants.

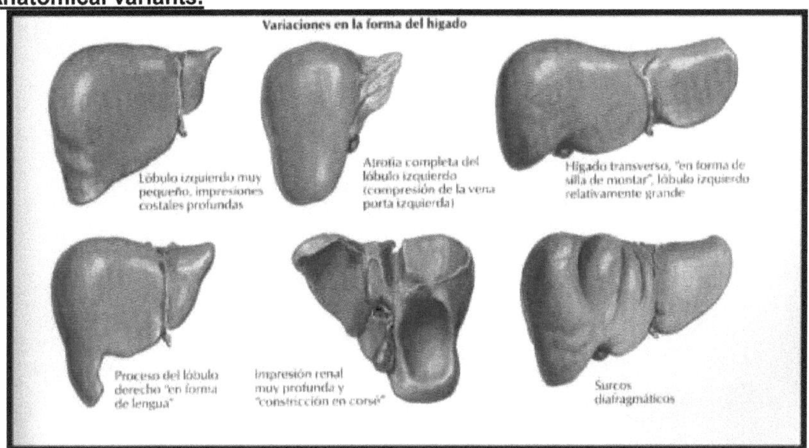

Normal appearance of the liver.

The liver shows a homogeneous structure, interrupted by the branches of the portal vein (PV), whose walls appear as linear echogenic structures. The thinner hepatic veins do not show echogenicity in their walls.

The inferior vena cava should be visualised in its intrahepatic tract and the aorta behind the liver.

Both lobes should be checked, as well as the caudate lobe, separated from the rest of the liver by a very echogenic line. Not to be confused with a 'T' image, especially in cases of liver cirrhosis.

The gall bladder, right kidney and pancreas should be identified. The normal echogenicity of the liver lies between the echogenicity of the pancreas (higher) and the spleen (lower).

IVC- inferior vena cava
RL- right hepatic lobe
LL- left hepatic lobe

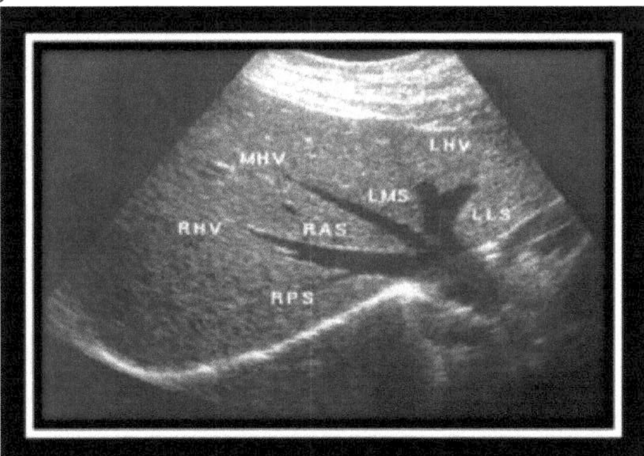

RHV- right hepatic vein MHV- middle hepatic vein LHV- left hepatic vein, separating lobules
And the segments.

The RHV separates the right posterior segment (RPS) from the right anterior segment (RAS).

The LHV separates the left medial segment (LMS) from the left lateral segment (LLS).

The MHV separates the right lobe from the left lobe.

Size and shape of the liver.

The right lobe is larger, although its shape and size is difficult to quantify. The cranio-caudal length of the LD at the level of the mid-clavicular Knea is approximately 15 cm.

When the ^gado is enlarged its edges become rounded although their shape and diameter vary greatly with body type.

There are wide variations in the size of the LI, which, when very small or elongated and in contact with the spleen, makes it difficult to examine.

CBD - common bile duct MPV - main portal vein Both are included within the hepatoduodenal ligament.
portal vein bifurcating into right and left branches

Sagittal section Transverse section
Branches of the portal vein Normal echogenicity of the liver

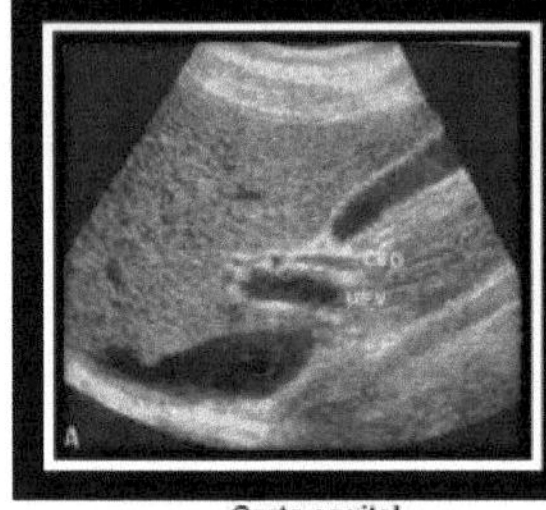

Corte sagital Corte transversal

CBD- conducto biliar común Vena porta que se bifurca
MPV- vena porta principal en la rama derecha e izquierda
Ambas incluidas dentro del
ligamento hepatoduodenal

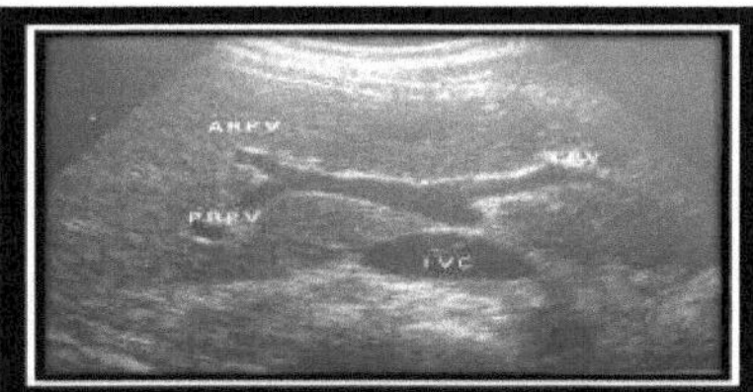

Ramas de la vena porta

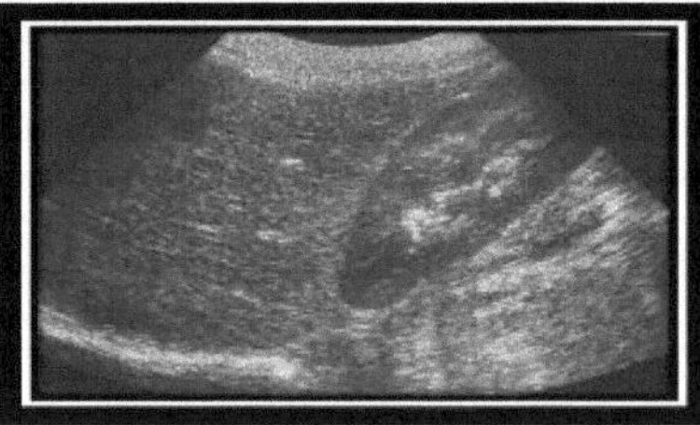

Ecogenicidad normal del Higado

<u>Pathological alterations.</u>
<u>(Diffuse hepatomegaly with homogeneous pattern).</u>
1   Fatty liver: fatty infiltration due to increased echogenicity.
2   CHF: There is dilatation of the hepatic veins; the IVC is not modified by respiration and can be seen, decreased echogenicity of the liver, cardiomegaly and pleural effusion.
3   Acute hepatitis: The liver parenchyma is hypoechogenic due to oedema of the hepatocytes, there is slight hepatomegaly and there is fibrosis and inflammation of the vessel walls.
4   Chronic hepatitis: The liver parenchyma is hyperechogenic, with decreased echogenicity of the walls of the PV branches.
5   Parasitism: Echinococcus alveolaris or multilocular, cystic image in which the parasite can be seen inside the cyst, may leave calcifications as a sequel.
<u>Pathological alterations.</u>
<u>(Diffuse inhomogeneous hepatomegaly).</u>
6   Absence of a defined mass: There is diffuse enhancement of echogenicity with loss of the reflective borders of the PV. There is poor visualisation of the deep structures of the liver.
-    Cirrhosis.
-    Chronic hepatitis.
-    Fatty liver.
2.- Presence of multiple echogenic masses:
-    **Macronodular cirrhosis:** there are areas of preserved liver tissue and altered vascular anatomy.
-    **Multiple abscesses:** There are internal echoes, with ill-defined borders.
-    **Metastases:** They can be hypo- or hyperechogenic, well or poorly demarcated. They cannot be differentiated from multinodular hepatocarcinoma.
-    **Lymphoma:** Multinodular hypoechogenic mass.
-    **Haematomas:** They may be hypoechogenic or hyperechogenic. Look for a history of trauma or treatment with anticoagulants.
<u>Pathological alterations.</u>
<u>(Small and retracted liver).</u>

Micronodular cirrhosis: small hyperechogenic liver, with distortion of the portal vein and hepatic veins. Associated with splenomegaly, ascites and varices. PV thrombosis must be ruled out.
<u>Pathological alterations.</u>
<u>(cystic lesion, normal or enlarged liver).</u>
1   Solitary cyst. They are rounded, almost always smaller than 3 cm.
2   Solitary cyst of irregular outline. Infested cyst or abscess.
3   Multiple cysts. Polycystic disease.
4   Complex cysts. Haemorrhage or infection.
5   Parasitic cyst. In a large number of cases, the larva can be seen inside the cyst.

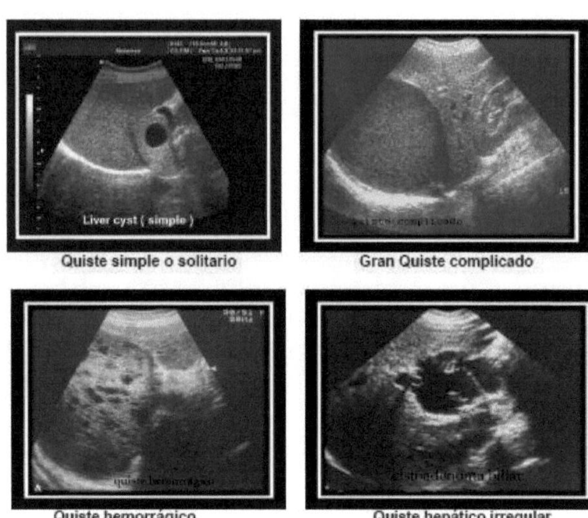

Quiste simple o solitario Gran Quiste complicado
Quiste hemorrágico Quiste hepático irregular

**Simple or solitary cyst Large Complicated cyst
Haemorrhagic cyst Irregular liver cyst**

Hepatic trauma.

Intrahepatic haematomas may appear hyperechogenic or hypoechogenic.

6   Subcapsular haematomas appear as anecogenic or complex areas between the liver capsule and the liver.

7   Extracapsular haematomas appear as anecogenous or complex areas surrounding the liver outside the capsule, similar to an abscess.

8   Bilomas are an accumulation of bile in or around the liver. The US appearance is similar to a haematoma.

Differential diagnosis of a hepatic mass (single solid mass).

1   Haemangioma. Hyperechogenic, well demarcated and proximal to the capsule. Has posterior sound enhancement without acoustic shadowing. When large they become mixed and simulate a malignant T.

2   Hepatocarcinoma. They can produce a homogeneous mass with poor echoes in the periphery, sometimes with central necrosis or they present as a diffuse mass with portal or hepatic infiltration.

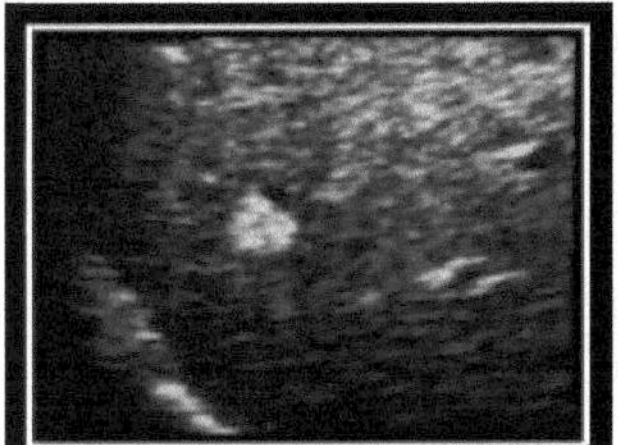

Masa ecogénica pequeña única.
Hemangioma de apariencia típica.

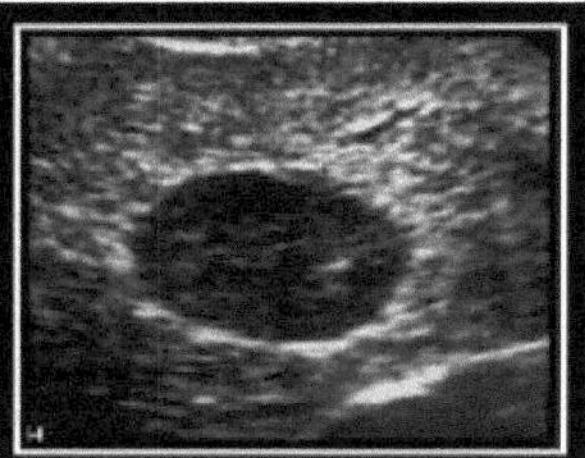

Centro granular hipoecogénico, fino anillo ecogénico. Hemangioma de apariencia atípica.

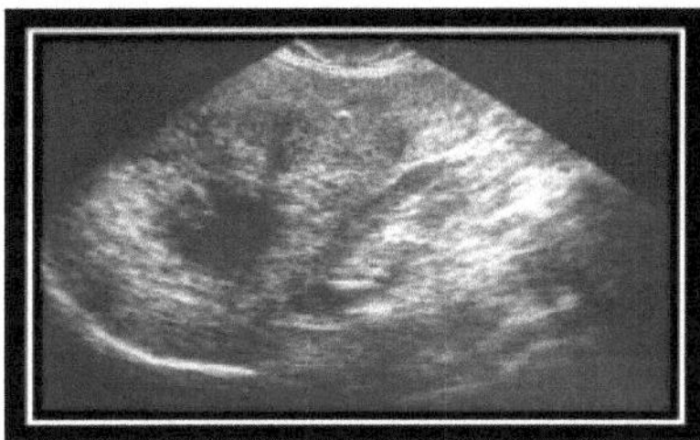

Corte sagital. Masa heterogénea y compleja en el lóbulo hepático derecho. Centro hipoecogénico (contenido líquido). Adenoma hemorrágico.

Single small echogenic mass.
Haemangioma of typical appearance.
Hypoechogenic granular centre, thin echogenic ring. Haemangioma of atypical appearance.
Sagittal section. Heterogeneous and complex mass in the right hepatic lobe. Hypoechogenic centre
(liquid content). Haemorrhagic adenoma.

Differential diagnosis of a hepatic mass (abscess).

Subphrenic and subhepatic abscess. It appears as an anecogenic area, well demarcated between the liver and the right hemidiaphragm. When it becomes chronic, the edges become irregular, septa appear and echoes are seen inside. Both subphrenic spaces should be examined. Sometimes the collection extends between the right liver and the right kidney.

Differential diagnosis of a hepatic mass. Abscesses).

1   Liver abscess. It is difficult to differentiate between bacterial abscess, amoebic or infected cyst. They may be single or multiple, hypoechogenic with thick walls with irregular contours and internal debris. The presence of gas can be identified.

2   Amoebic abscess. Initially they are isoechogenic and not visible, or echogenic with poorly defined borders, later they are well delimited and the internal material shows fine echoes. When they heal they may become calcified.

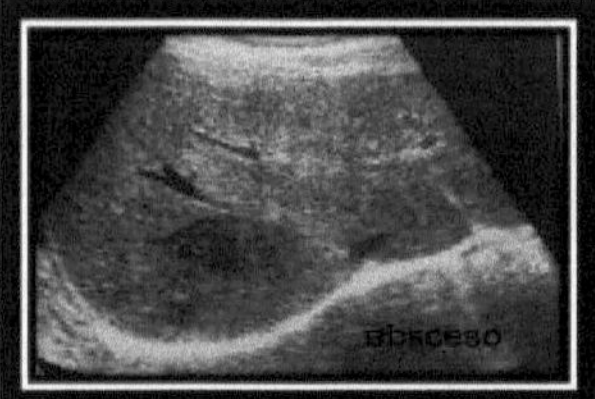

Imagen transversal del lóbulo derecho
Mostrándose un sutil "efecto de masa"
Hipoecogénico y pobremente definido

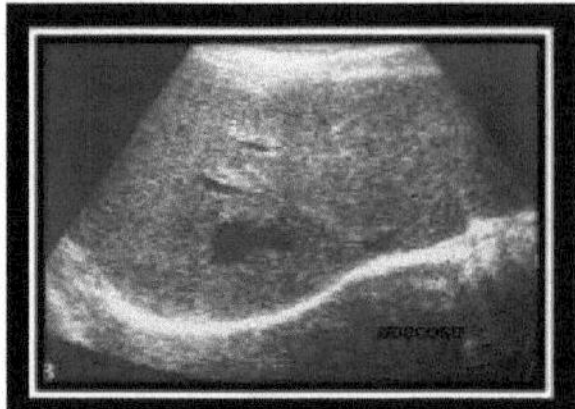

(24 horas)

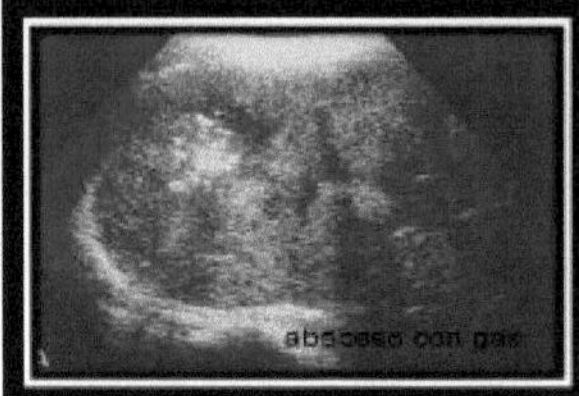

Masa hepática mal definida con
innumerables focos pequeños
ecogénicos brillantes en su interior.
Absceso hepático con gas secundario.

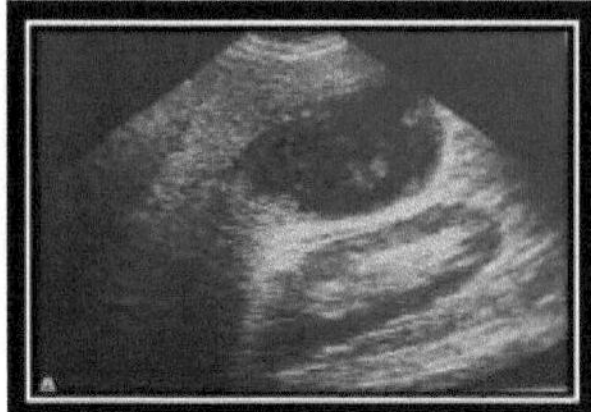

Masa hipoecogénica, márgenes mal
definidos que abomba la cápsula
hepática con ecos internos.
Absceso hepático piógeno.

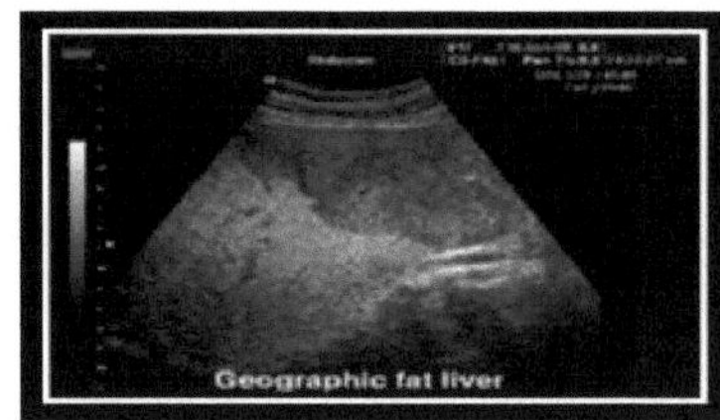

Masa hiperecogénica con bordes irregulares que no alteran la vena porta.
Esteatosis Hepática.

Cross-sectional image of the right lobe showing a subtle "mass effect" Hypoechogenic and poorly defined.
(24 hours)
Ill-defined hepatic mass with innumerable small bright echogenic foci inside. Hepatic abscess with secondary gas.
Hypoechogenic mass, poorly defined margins abutting the liver capsule with internal echoes. Pyogenic liver abscess.
Hyperechogenic mass with irregular borders that do not alter the portal vein. Hepatic steatosis.

Chapter 3

Ultrasound of the gallbladder and bile ducts.
Indications for Ultrasound of the Gallbladder and Biliary Tract.
1   Dyspepsia.
2   Pain in CSD. Gall bladder colic or cholecystitis.
3   .- fctero.
4   HD Mass.
5   Peptic ulcer symptoms.
6   Indication for lithotripsy.
Anatomy of the Vesphcula.
In CS, the vesicle has a peripheral appearance, is anecogenic, and is no larger than 4 cm. Its position is very variable, ranging from a very high position in the HD to a position in the FI. If it cannot be seen in its normal position, it is necessary to check the whole abdomen or repeat the examination on another day. The thickness of the bladder wall on CT ranges from 1 to 3 mm. When the bladder is examined 30, 45, 60 minutes after a fatty meal, the degree of emptying can be determined.

In a sagittal or longitudinal section, the gallbladder should measure 8 to 11 cm in its largest or longitudinal diameter, and the antero-posterior diameter is half of the longitudinal diameter. Its walls measure up to 3 mm when fasting, but in a distended gallbladder its walls can measure up to 1 mm. In order to measure the functioning of the gallbladder it is necessary to evaluate the interior of this organ, if it is not occupied, it is done in the following way: a volume of the organ must be taken on an empty stomach and another post-fasting, after administering a meal rich in fat (which can be anything from a small teaspoonful of oil to a breakfast containing this element, the fat), once this action has been carried out, wait 30, 45 to 60 minutes to take a second volume, which must have decreased to 60% of the initial volume to confirm that it is functioning adequately.

Normal anatomy of the bile ducts.
Intrahepatic BVs are not always visible, appearing as thin-walled, tubular, anechogenic structures.

The common hepatic duct is located in front and to the right of the VP and should not exceed 5 mm. The choledochus is variable in size, but should not exceed 9 mm, sometimes measuring up to 1 cm, but the diameter we are talking about is the antero-posterior, longitudinal section of the duct.

The calibre of the choledochus varies with age, especially in elderly and cholecystectomised patients, but in the latter case it should not exceed 10-12 mm.

❖   It is located on the posterior caudal surface of the ^gado where it separates the right lobe from the left lobe.

❖   The vesicle is an elongated sac (longitudinal diameter is twice its transverse diameter and its wall measures approximately 3 mm).

❖   The rtstic is a thin, tortuous duct, less than 3mm in diameter, in which thin echogenic septa can be visualised, corresponding to the folds of the duct.

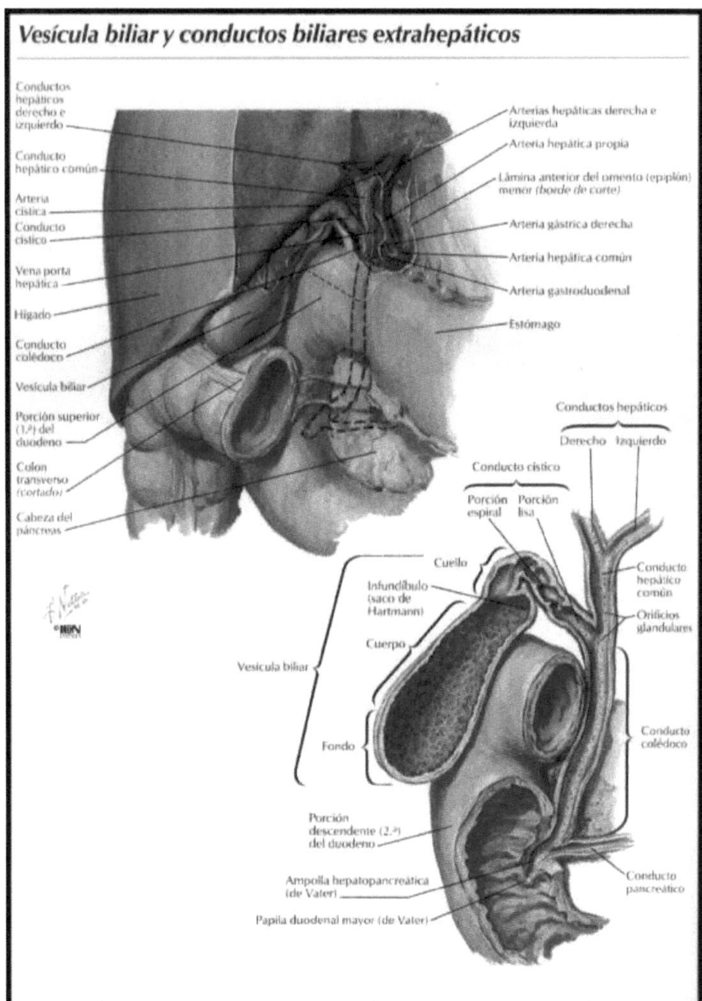

Normal gallbladder. Preparation of the patient.

This study should be performed on an empty stomach and in some cases to assess the gall bladder it is necessary to

The test should be performed after an 8-hour fast and after eating a high-fat meal.

In urgent cases or for complementary US studies without specific indication, it can be performed without the 8-hour fasting period.

Ultrasound technique of the bladder and bile ducts.

The entire HS should be examined in the supine and sometimes left oblique position with a 3.5 or 5 MHz transducer.

Perform transverse, longitudinal (*deep inspiration*), and intercostal sections, the latter useful in children, elderly and uncooperative patients.

Normal variants of Vesfcula.

1   Biloculate vesfcula.
2   Congenital folds or vesicular kinks.

3   Tabication (if complete it is often associated with bile stasis, cholelithiasis and cholecystitis).
4   Double vesicle with two dstic ducts (very rare).
Pre- and post-pandral bladder.
Pathological alterations I. (No visualisation of the Vesphcula).
1   The patient is not fasting.
2   The vesicle is ectopic in location.
3   Hypoplastic vesicle or vesicular agenesis.
4   Scleroatrophic vesfcula, usually with lithiasis.
5   Cholecystectomised patient.
Pathological alterations II (distended bladder).
The bladder is considered distended when it has a transverse diameter greater than 4 cm, in case of doubts in vesicular emptying it will allow to determine the degree of vesicular contraction.
1   Dehydrated patient.
2   Low-fat diets or E-V nutrition. Prolonged.
3   Patients immobilised for periods of time.
4   Obstruction of the duodenum or choledochus, (lithiasis, lymph nodes, parasites, tumours, etc.).
5   Cholecystitis. Thickening of the wall above 5 mm and pain on transducer pressure. A perivesicular anechogenic ring (perforation) can be seen, lithiasis is almost always present.
In cholecystitis, there may be no lithiasis and the gallbladder may not be distended.
Pathological alterations III (Presence of intravesicular echoes).
1   Mobile echoes with SA.
- Lithiasis. They produce bright echoes regardless of the degree of calcification. They may be single or multiple. There may or may not be alterations of the wall.
The finding of a lithiasis does not always justify the symptoms.
BV stones are not easy to identify.
2   Mobile echoes without SA.
-    Lithiasis smaller than the beam diameter of our US equipment.
-    Thick bile. Associated with chronic obstruction or infection.
-    Blood clots.
-    Membranes of a hydatid cyst.
-    Parasites.
3   Internal non-moving echoes with SA.
-    Impacted lithiasis.
-    Calcification of the vesicular wall.
4   Non-moving internal echoes without SA.
-    Polyp. Occasionally the peduncle may be visible, not modified by changes in position.
-    Septum or septum.
-    Biliary mud.
-    Malignant tumour.
Pathological alterations V. (Thickening of the vesicular wall).
1   Diffuse thickening.
1   Acute cholecystitis.
2   Chronic cholecystitis.
3   Decreased serum albumin, often associated with CH.
4   ICC.
5   IRC.
6   Malignant myeloma (MM).

7   Hyperplastic cholecystitis or adenomyomatosis.
8   Acute hepatitis.
9   Lymphoma.
2   <u>Localised thickening.</u>
1   Wall folds. They change with changes in the patient's position and during the examination.
2   Polyps.
3   Carcinoma. A localised, solid, intravesicular mass that grows towards the lumen and may involve or infiltrate the ^-gland.
Pathological alterations (small vesicle).
1   The patient is not fasting.
2   Chronic cholecystitis. The examination should be repeated after 6 to 8 hours fasting or after three days on a low-fat diet. Small vesicle. Icteric syndrome I.
US can differentiate between obstructive and non-obstructive fcterus, but cannot always determine the cause.
The technique varies somewhat in these patients:
It is advisable to start the examination in CS or Oblique to identify the IVC and the PV in order to locate the extrahepatic BVs which are located descending from the ^gut at an angle in front of the PV. It is advisable to move the patient in different positions.
Intrahepatic ducts are best located in the left lobe, in deep inspiration and when pathological they appear as irregularly branched structures, close to the branches of the PV.
Bile duct dilatation. Obstructive jaundice.
It is important to assess the bladder, because if it is distended, the obstruction is located below the hepatorttic confluent. There are exceptions to this rule, because if the bladder is scleroatrophic, it is not distended.
If the extrahepatic ducts are dilated but not the intrahepatic ducts and in the presence of a persistent jaundice, we must think of CH or an obstruction of the extrahepatic BV.
Examination of the pancreas, especially the pancreatic head and the pancreaticobiliary duodenal confluent is important in these cases.

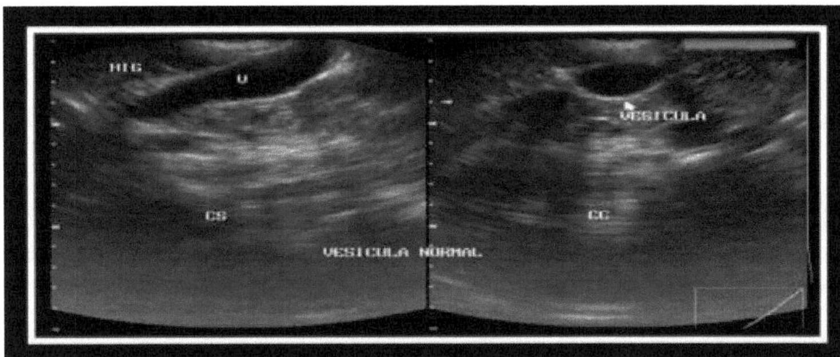

Sagittal section

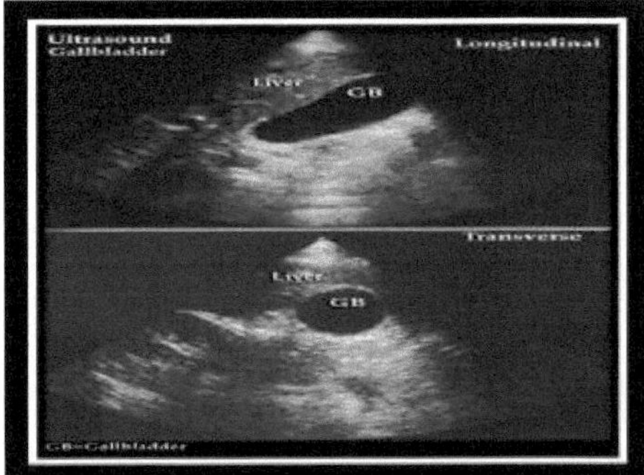

Corte transverso

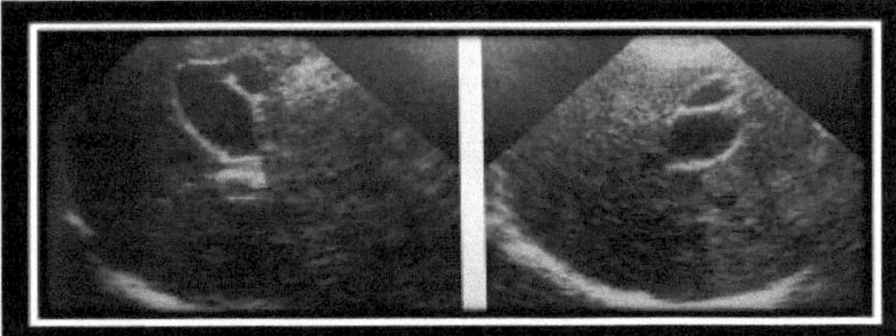

Vesícula en gorro frigio

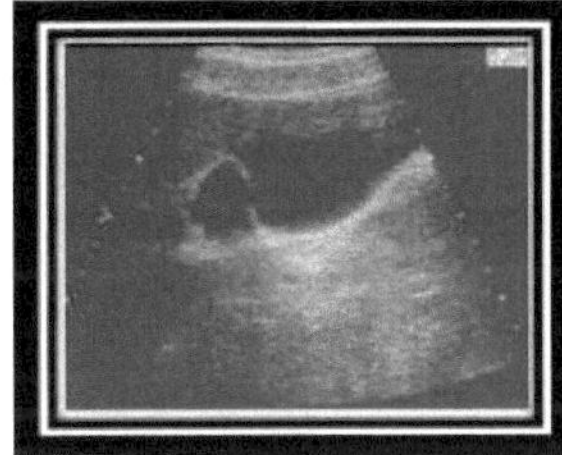

Vesícula con septo

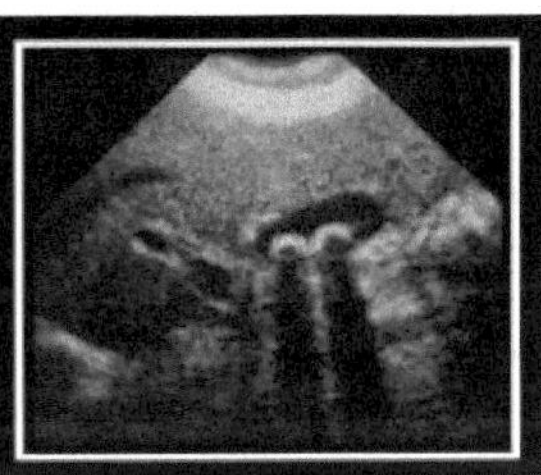

Litiasis vesicular

Transverse cut
Vesfcula in Phrygian cap
Vesicle with septum Gall bladder stones

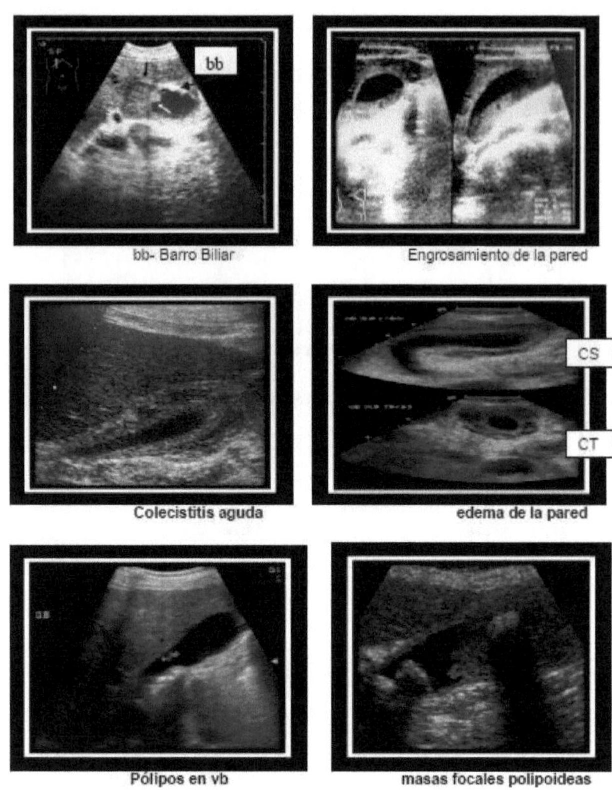

bb- Barro Biliar

Engrosamiento de la pared

Colecistitis aguda

edema de la pared

Pólipos en vb

masas focales polipoideas

bb- Biliary Mud Thickening of the bile wall
Acute cholecystitis wall oedema
Polyps in vb focal polypoid masses

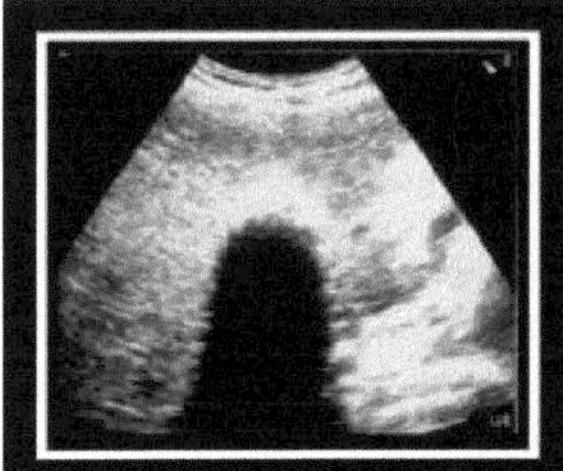 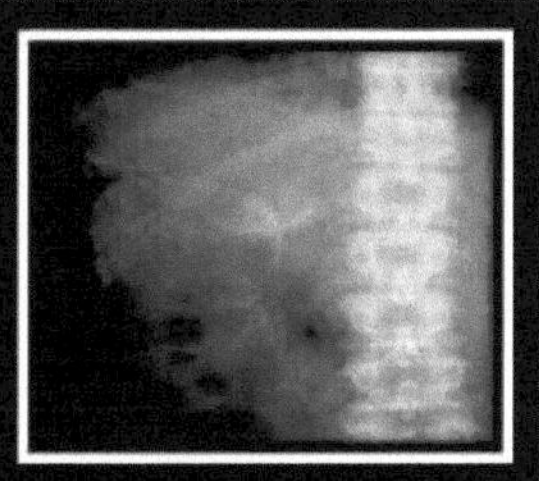

Dilatación de la vía biliar: vesícula en porcelana

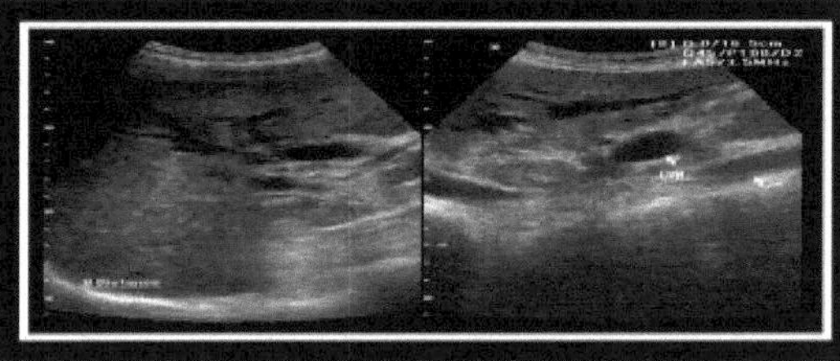

Lesiones obstructivas: litiasis coledociana

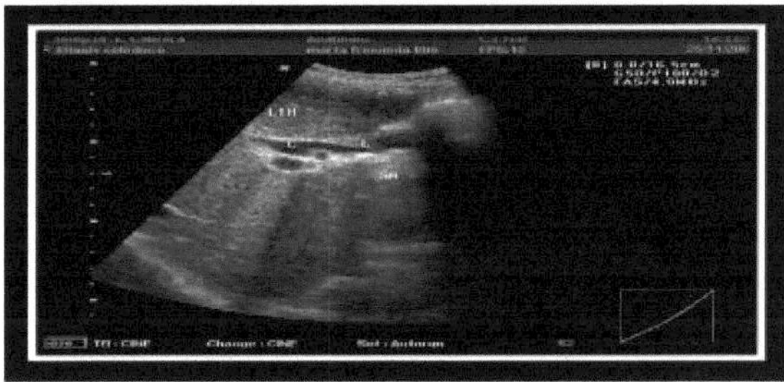

Múltiples cálculos en el conducto biliar

Bile duct dilatation: porcelain vesfcule
Obstructive lesions: choledochal lithiasis
Multiple stones in the bile duct

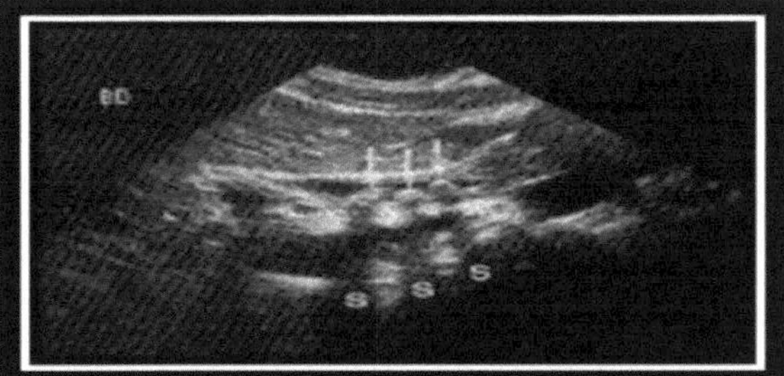

Chapter 4

Ultrasound of the Spleen.

Indications for Spleen US.
1   Splenomegaly.
2   T mass in upper hemiabdomen.
3   Closed traumas.
4   Pain in CSI.
5   fctero with anaemia.
6   Suspected subphrenic abscess.
7   Hydatid disease.
8   Ascites.
9   Lymphoma or leukaemia.
10 Suspected portal hypertension.

Preparation and Technique.
The study is performed with the patient in the supine decubitus position and giving an obliquity of 30 degrees on the right side.
Oblique intercostal and transverse slices are made over the IH, as well as sagittal slices in deep inspiration.

Normal ultrasonographic anatomy of the spleen.
The normal pattern of the spleen is uniform and homogeneous, less echogenic than the liver and more echogenic than the kidney. It should not exceed 15 cm in its major axis or close to the size of the left kidney.
Spleen US should be identified:
1   The splenic hilum.
2   The splenic veins.
3   The left kidney.
4   Hepatic left lobe.
5   The pancreas.

Pathological alterations of the spleen.
(Diffuse splenomegaly).
1   Parasitism.
2   Sicklemia.
3   Metabolic disease.
4   Lymphoma. Hypoechogenic nodules may be seen.
5   Infectious processes (mononucleosis).
6   AIDS.

Pathological alterations of the spleen.
(Well-defined cystic lesions).
Cystic lesions may occur with or without splenomegaly.
1   Polycystic diseases.
2   Congenital cysts.
3   Hydatid cysts.
4   Haematoma.
Splenic cysts can be:
1   Primary congenital (true cysts) are non-parasitic cysts.
2   Pseudocysts (most frequently of post-traumatic origin).
3   Polycystic (hereditary) disease.
4   Hydatid cyst (less common in the spleen, may calcify its wall).

Pathological alterations of the spleen.
(ill-defined cystic lesion, abscesses).
Abscesses are more frequent in immunocompromised patients or patients with bacterial endocarditis.

Four categories are defined:
-   Pyogenic embolic abscesses.
-   Post-traumatic infectious.
-   Sickle cell abscess.
-   Abscesses by extension from neighbouring organs.
The ultrasound aspect of abscesses:
-   Septate collections or collections with necrotic material that may simulate a hydatid disease.
-   Small nodular lesions.
-   Collections with gaseous content with highly reflective echoes.
-   Subphrenic abscess, non-echoic or complex mass above the spleen (diaphragmatic hypomobility and pleural effusion).
-   Hypo- or anechoic collections similar to cysts or haematomas in liquefaction.

<u>Pathological alterations of the spleen.</u>
<u>(Calcifications).</u>
Calcifications may be related to:
-   Inflammatory granulomas, TB, Histoplasmosis.
-   Chronic haematoma.
-   Calcification of the splenic artery.
-   Splenic artery aneurysm.

<u>Pathological alterations of the spleen.</u>
<u>(Intrasplenic mass).</u>
A splenic mass may occur with or without splenomegaly.
1   Lymphoma. Hypoechogenic mass. Primary lymphoma in the spleen is very rare, being more frequent the NHL variety.
2   Metastases. Hypo- or hyperechogenic nodule or mass.
3   Inflammatory granulomas due to TB or fungi. Hyperechogenic masses with calcifications.

<u>Pathological alterations of the spleen.</u>
<u>(Smdrome febrile).</u>
Subphrenic abscess, mass without echoes or may present in a complex form above the spleen with little mobility of the diaphragm.

<u>Pathological alterations of the spleen.</u>
<u>(Closed abdominal trauma).</u>
1   Injury to the spleen. Intrasplenic or subphrenic free kyphosis with loss of spleen contours.
2   Subsplenic haematoma. There is splenomegaly and an anechogenic or mixed area.
3   Chronic haematoma. Intrasplenic echogenic mass, sometimes calcified.
4   Traumatic cysts. Anechogenic or complex mass with irregular borders.

<u>Pathological alterations of the spleen.</u>
<u>(Portal hypertension).</u>
The splenic vein is more than 13 mm in diameter and does not change with respiration. Collateral vessels can be seen and the entire spleno-portal axis should always be examined.

<u>Pathological alterations of the spleen.</u>
<u>(Tumours).</u>
-   Angiosarcomas.
-   Malignant haemangioendotheliomas.
They are rare tumours and may present as large, highly vascularised echogenic masses.

<u>**Pathological alterations of the spleen.**</u>
<u>**(Metastasis).**</u>
Metastases are rare in the spleen, but carcinoma of the breast, lung and melanoma of the testis can frequently metastasise to the spleen.
They can be single or multiple, small or large, are hypoechoic with the appearance of target shooting, and can often be seen as echogenic images with no RP or very poor RP.
<u>**Pathological alterations of the spleen.**</u>
<u>**(Splenic infarcts).**</u>
Most often embolic in cause.
In the early period, the spleen may appear normal.
Triangular peripheral zone with low amplitude echoes.
Healing phase: echogenic due to fibrosis, calcifications, cystic.
Complications: Infection, haemorrhage, pseudocyst formation.
<u>**Pathological alterations of the spleen.**</u>
<u>**(Trauma).**</u>
The most frequently injured organ in blunt abdominal trauma. Associated with rib fractures.
Pleural effusion may be present.
Spontaneous rupture may occur in a pathological spleen.
Classification:
Contusion or laceration without capsular rupture
Parenchymal laceration with capsular rupture
Lesion of the hilum vessels
In spleen contusions:
- No alteration (20% are not clinically obvious).
- Parenchyma not homogeneous in appearance.
- Laceration with haematoma: depending on the stage.

Evolution:
- Return to normal, residual scarring or pseudocysts. Subcapsular laceration: subcapsular collection.
- With capsular rupture: free blood in the peritoneum surrounding the spleen or in the recesses of the peritoneal cavity.
- Spontaneous rupture.

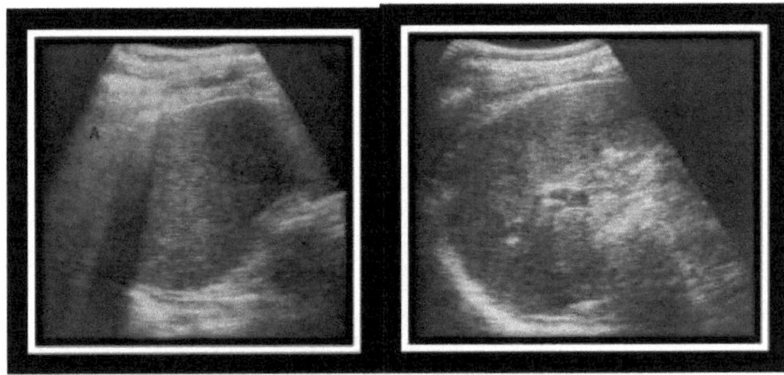

Exploración esplénica

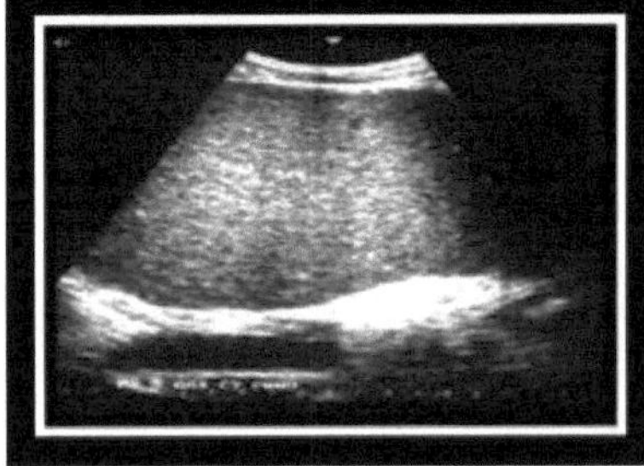

Esplenomegalia en hipertensión portal

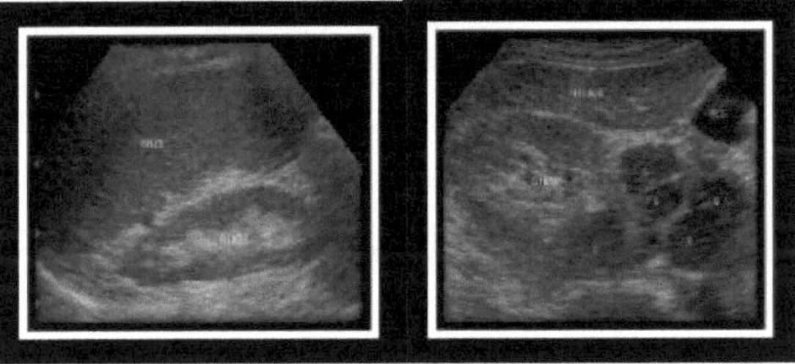

Splenic exploration
Splenomegaly in portal hypertension

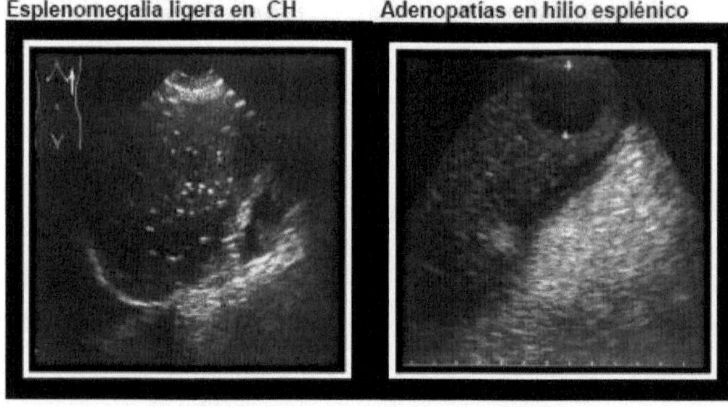

Granulomas calcificados   Absceso esplénico

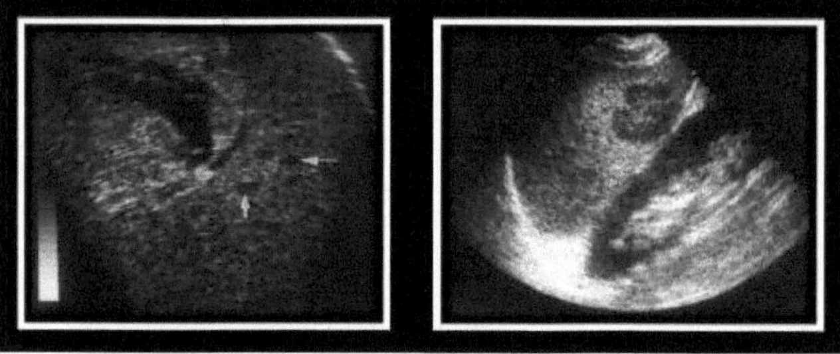

Mild splenomegaly in CH Adenopathies in splenic hilum
Calcified granulomas Splenic abscess
AIDS patient. Microabscesses Splenic lymphoma.

Chapter 5

Ultrasound of the Pancreas.

Indications for US of the Pancreas.

1   Acute or chronic pain in the epigastrium.
2   .- fctero.
3   Tumour in H.A. S.
4   Feverish syndrome, with abdominal discomfort.
5   Suspicion of malignant process.
6   History of acute or chronic pancreatitis.
7   In complications of acute pancreatitis.
8   Polycystic diseases.
9   Direct abdominal trauma.

Preparation and Technique.

Fasting patient, lying supine, 3.5 or 5 MHz transducers are used.

Transverse cuts are made in the epigastrium from the subcostal region to the umbilicus and longitudinal cuts in the medial and parasagittal lhea preferably in deep inspiration.

If there is intestinal gas that makes visualisation difficult, it is recommended that the patient drinks 3 to 4 glasses of water.

In CT scans, the junction of the EV with the SM behind the pancreas must be identified. It is necessary to try to identify the head and the uncinate process that are somewhat

and are located between the IVC and the PV.

In the LCs and towards the right side, the IVC and the PV must be identified as the head of the pancreas is situated anteriorly. On the left side, the Ao and the AM must be identified in close relation to the body of the pancreas.

Normal ultrasonographic appearance of the pancreas.

The normal pancreas has a homogeneous, liver-like echogenicity with smooth contours. The following structures should always be identified: Ao, IVC, SMA, EV, gastric wall and choledochus. Especially the SMA and the EV.

There are wide variations in the size and shape of the normal pancreas:

-   Average head diameter: 2.8 cm.

-   Average body diameter: less than 2 cm.

-   Average tail diameter: 2.5 cm.

-   Duct diameter: not to exceed 2 mm.

Normal pancreas.

Normal variants of the pancreas.

1   Prominent tail: may be larger than the body and may lend itself to confusion with a tumour mass.

As many slices as possible should be made in order to visualise the pancreatic head from different angles and planes.

2   Asymmetric lipomatosis: there are focal hypoechogenic areas which, when compared with the rest of the echogenic glandular structure, can lead to false diagnoses.

Pathological alterations of the Pancreas I.

(Small pancreas).

1   Elderly patients. Increases its echogenicity due to fat infiltration.
2   Chronic pancreatitis. It is irregularly hypoechogenic and inhomogeneous.

Pathological alterations of the pancreas II.
(Diffuse enlargement of the pancreas).
Acute pancreatitis. With normal or decreased echogenicity. Acute pancreatitis can present in four ways:
- Oedematous.
- Phlegm.
- Haemorrhagic.
- Necrotising.

2.- Acute chronic pancreatitis. With irregular hyperechogenicity.
Di rectum signs of pancreatitis.
Indirect signs of pancreatitis.
Pancreatic and peripancreatic collections.
Pancreatic abscess.
It is a collection of necrotic pancreatic tissue mixed with blood and pus, the most frequent causative germ being E. coli. Coli. It occurs most frequently in necrotising pancreatitis and postoperative pancreatitis.
In its early stages, US offers little information to make a diagnosis of pancreatic abscess. In the acute and subacute phases, the appearance is indistinguishable from oedematous or phlegmonous pancreatitis or may be mistaken for a sterile liquid collection.
Pathological alterations of the pancreas.
(Localised non-cyst enlargement).
1   Pancreatic tumour. Usually hypoechogenic with respect to the intestine or the rest of the pancreas.
Pancreatic lymphoma.
Primary lymphoma is very rare, although in autopsies of patients with lymphoma the pancreas is involved in 35%, especially in Burkitt's lymphoma.
Peripancreatic lymph nodes are most often involved, intrapancreatic masses are not uncommon.
On ultrasound they are indistinguishable from other pancreatic T types.
The pancreas may appear diffusely thickened and of low echogenicity, but it is also enlarged by the presence of multiple small hypoechoic nodules.
The existence of alterations in the abdominal organs and intra- or retroperitoneal lymph nodes, or knowledge of a previous diagnosis of lymphoma, helps in the interpretation of the images and in making the diagnosis.
Pancreatic metastases.
Most pancreatic metastases occur via the haematogenous route, with direct invasion being less common.
They can originate from melanoma, carcinoma of the lung, breast, ovary, testicle, prostate, liver or kidney, as well as from sarcoma.
It is also possible to infiltrate neighbouring T's (stomach, colon and kidney).
Pathological alterations of the pancreas IV.
(predominantly cystic localised enlargement).
2   True cysts. Without echoes and thin-walled. Single or multiple.
3   Abscesses or haematomas. Complex masses associated with pancreatitis.
4   Pseudocysts caused by trauma or pancreatitis. At first they are complex and then become thin-walled echolucent, if infected, internal echoes appear. They can have any location in the abdomen.
5   Pancreatic cystadenoma. Multitabular cystic masses with solid components.
6   Hydatid cyst.

<u>**Pathological alterations of the pancreas V.**</u>
<u>**(Pancreatic calcifications).**</u>
US is not the method of choice with CT being of much greater value in the detection of pancreatic calcifications.
1   Chronic pancreatitis.
2   Calculations in the pancreatic duct.
3   Calculations in the distal portion of the choledochus.
<u>**Pathological alterations of the pancreas VI.**</u>
<u>**(Pancreatic duct dilatation).**</u>
The normal calibre of the pancreatic duct is 2 mm and it is best visualised in cross-sections at the level of the body. Its walls are smooth and its contents are echolucent. Dilatation may be due to:
1   Tumour of the head of the pancreas.
2   Tumour in the ampulla of Vater.
3   Calculations in the main pancreatic duct.
4   Calculations in the intrapancreatic ducts.
5   Chronic pancreatitis.
6   Postoperative narrowing.

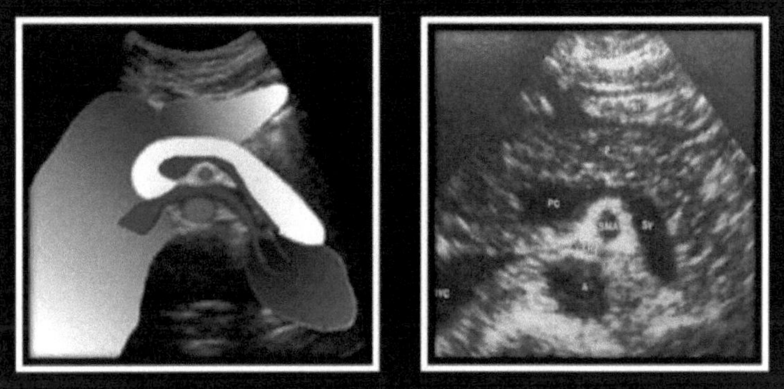

Cross section at the level of the epigastrium

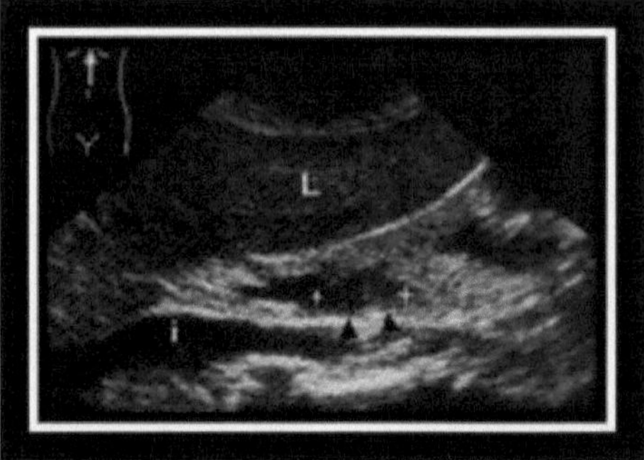

Sagittal section in the epigastrium

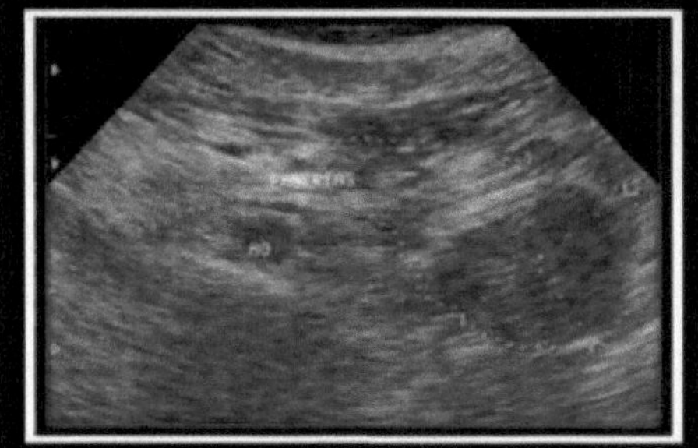

Pancreatic tail tumour

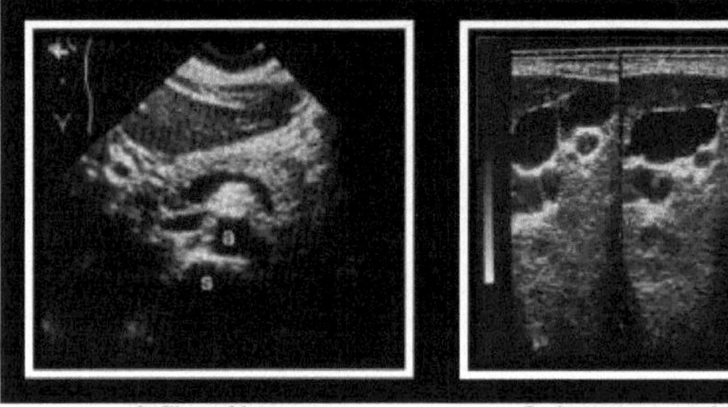

Infiltración grasa   Quistes pancreáticos

Fatty infiltration Pancreatic cysts

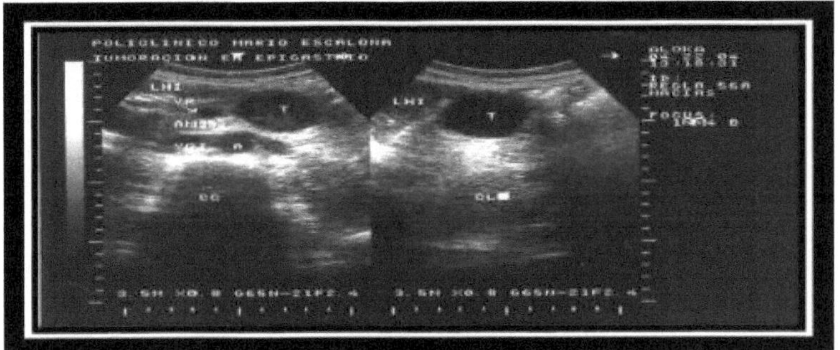

Tumor del Páncreas

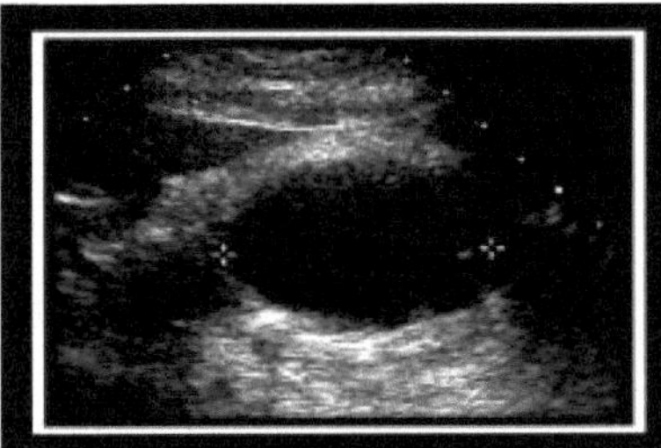

Pseudoquiste simple

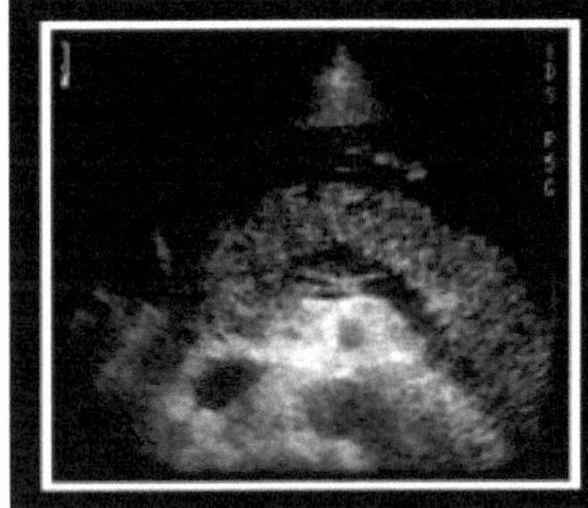

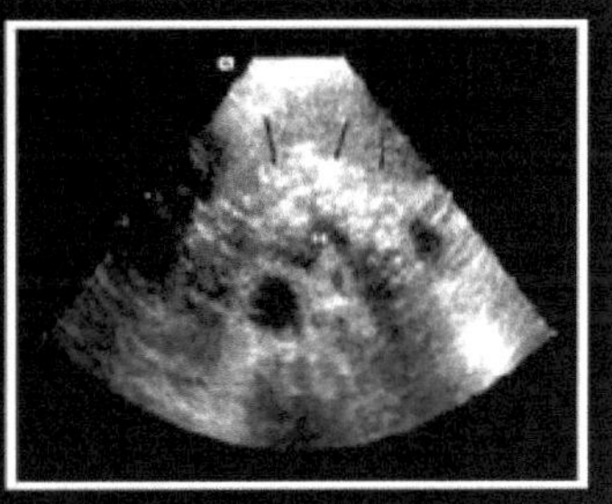

Páncreas aumentado
difusamente

Pancreatitis crónica
con cálculo en su interior

Pancreatic Tumour
Simple pseudocyst
Diffusely enlarged pancreas
Chronic pancreatitis with calculus in its interior

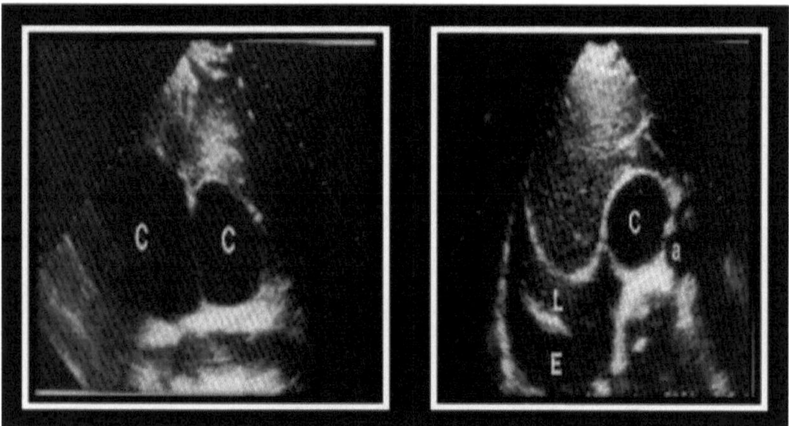

Large, complicated pseudocyst extending into the
Chest fluid in the right chest cavity with collapsed lung.

Chapter 6

Renoureteral Ultrasound.

Indications for Renoureteral US.
1   Renal or ureteral pain.
2   Suspicion of a renal or adrenal mass.
3   Non-functioning rhinon in the descending urogram.
4   Haematuria.
5   Recurrent renal infection.
6   Blunt trauma of the abdomen.
7   Suspected polycystic disease.
8   Fever of unknown aetiology.
9   Parasitic disease.
10   Uncontrolled high blood pressure.
11   Evaluation of renal transplantation and its possible complications.

Preparation and Technique I.
Renoureteral US does not require preparation unless the bladder is examined.

The patient lies supine, longitudinal and transverse slices are made by moving the transducer up and down and back and forth. Sometimes it is necessary to place the patient in the prone position by placing a pillow between the bed and the patient's abdomen. When studying the DR, the abdomen is used as an acoustic window, with the patient taking a deep breath in. The patient can be placed in the left lateral decubitus position to better study the DR and in the right decubitus position to better study the RI, sometimes it is necessary to perform the study by placing the patient in a standing or sitting position.

The renoureteral US study is comparative, taking into account the variations in size, echogenicity and contours of both kidneys.

3.5 or 5 MHz transducers are used, adjusting the gains of the equipment.

Normal anatomy of the kidney.
1   Length: 9-12 cm.
2   Width: 4-6 cm.
3   Thickness: greater than 3.5 cm.
4   In the child, the kidneys are about 4 cm long and 2 cm wide.
5   The central portion is echogenic, occupying one third of the kidney.
6   The renal pyramids can be seen as hypoechogenic areas in the medullary portion of the kidney, surrounded by the cortical which is more echogenic.

In renoureteral US, the following structures should be identified:
1   The renal capsule. Smooth, shiny, echogenic lhea surrounding the kidney.
2   The cortical is less echogenic than the ^gado and more echogenic than the pyramids.
3   The renal medulla containing the pyramids.
4   The renal sinus in the internal position of the kidney and with great echogenicity (fat, collecting system and blood vessels).
5   The ureters. They are best visualised in coronal section.
6   The renal vessels.

Renal malformations.
1   A normal rhinum with a genesic rhinum.
2   Rinon digenesic.
3   Hypoplastic rhinon.
4   Rinon badly rotated.
5   Renal ectopia (thoracic, lumbar, sacral variant).
7   Crossed renal ectopia (with and without fusion).
8   Rinon in cake.

9   Horseshoe rhinon.
10   Rinon supernumerary
Pathological alterations of the Rhinon.
(Renal absence).
The search for and localisation of the rhinum should be insisted upon. Absence of the rhinum is accompanied by compensatory hypertrophy of the single rhinum. Ectopia must be ruled out, but very small kidneys are difficult to visualise (less than 2 cm thick and less than 4 cm long).
Renal pathologies.
(Obstruction of the excretory system).
1   Hydronephrosis or hydroureter.
2   Obstruction of the ureteropelvic junction.
3   Renal lithiasis.
4   Ureteral lithiasis.
5   Adenomegaly.
6   Tumours.
7   . - Hydronephrosis or hydroureter.
Renal pathologies.
(Infectious processes).
1   Pyonephrosis or pyonephrosis.
2   Chronic pyelonephritis.
3   Renal abscess.

Benign renal expansive processes.
1   Qusticos.
-    Simple cortical cyst.
-    Parapelvic cysts.
-    Extraparenchymal cysts.
-    Complicated cyst.
-    Polycystic disease.
-    Childhood polycystic disease.
2   Solids.
-    Angiomyolipoma or renal hamartoma.
-    Oncocytoma.
-    Haematoma.

<u>**Malignant renal expansive processes.**</u>
1   Hypernephroma.
2   Sarcoma.
3   Willms' tumour.
4   Transitional cell carcinoma.
5   Lymphomas (NHL, HL).
6   Leukaemias.

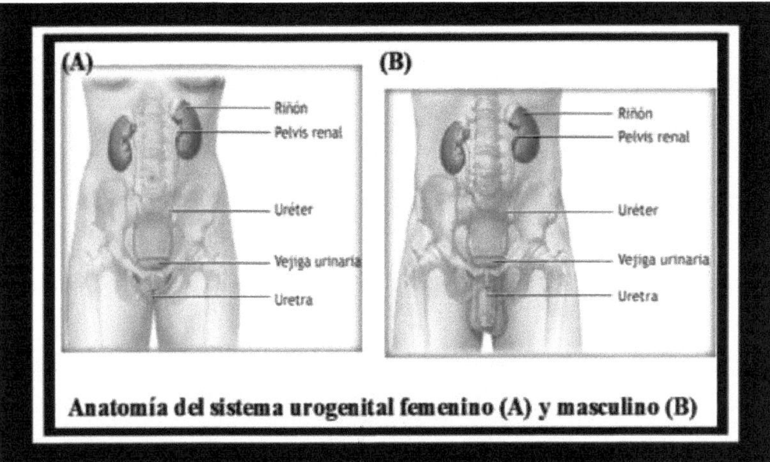

Sagittal section to the right hypochondrium

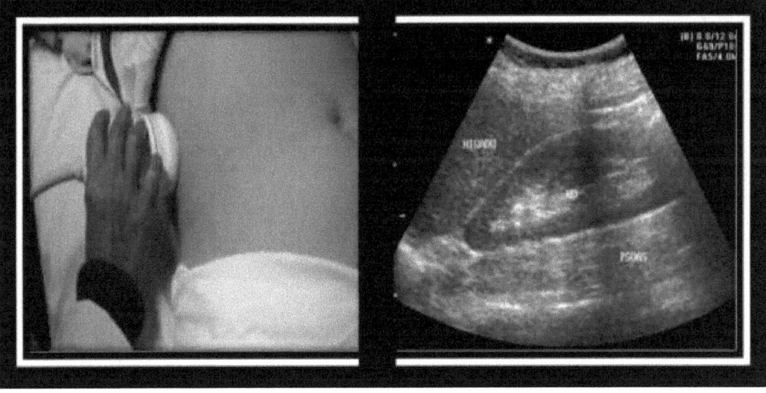

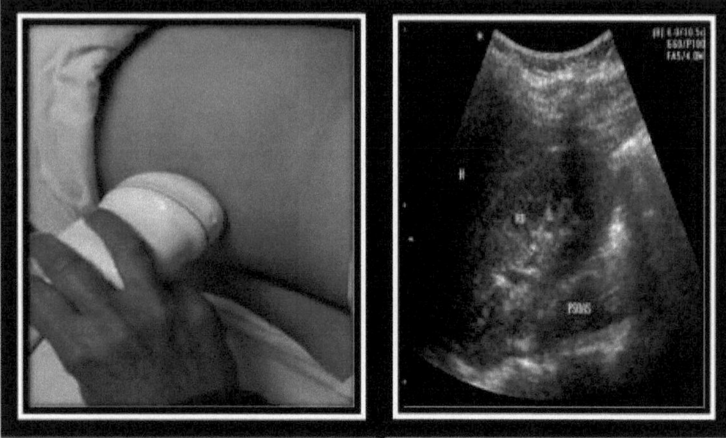

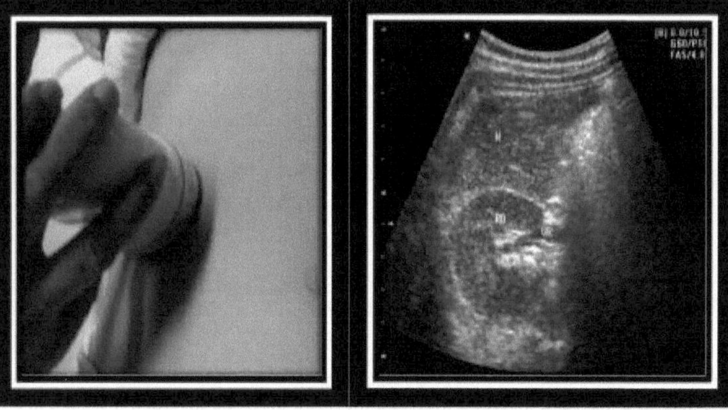

Posterior section with eppl right oblique patient
CCoronal orte orte orte coronal nal to the right hypochondrochondrial right hypochondrium

NORMAL DIMENSIONS OF BOTH KIDNEYS

The liver and spleen can be used as acoustic windows for the evaluation of the kidneys. The diameters should be measured:

- Length 10 to 13 cm
- Width 4.9 to 6.4
- Antero posterior 3.9 to 8.1 cm

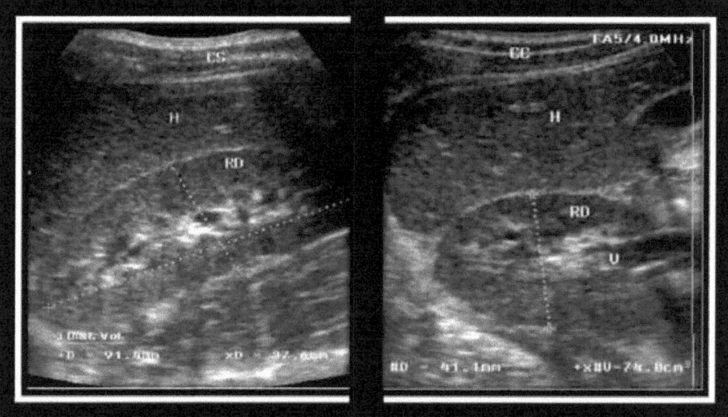

Congenital abnormalities and anatomical variants renal agenesis

On ultrasound, one of the kidneys is not visualised and the opposite renal cell is occupied by a loop which may simulate a pathological kidney.
The opposite kidney appears enlarged.

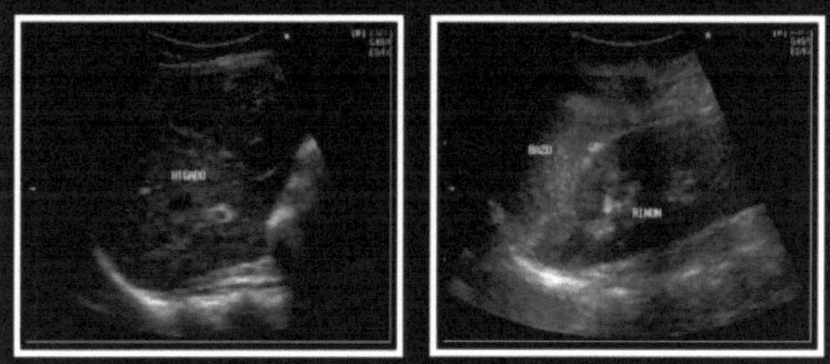

Hypoplastic rhinon

In this ultrasound the kidney is small but normal looking. It is very difficult to differentiate it from an atrophic kidney.
Foetal lobulation

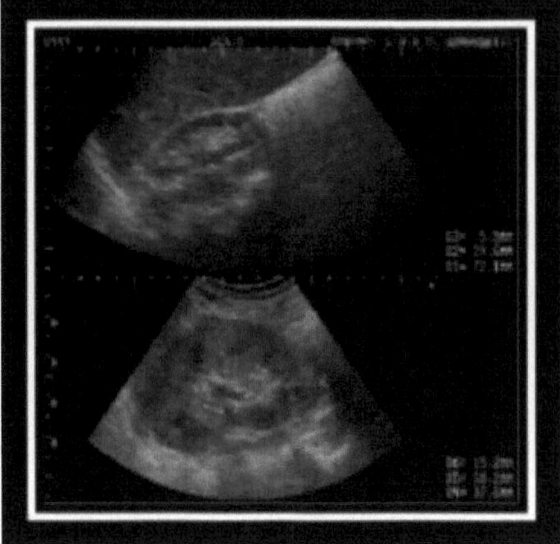

Lobulación fetal

On ultrasound, it presents with deposits on the renal surface.

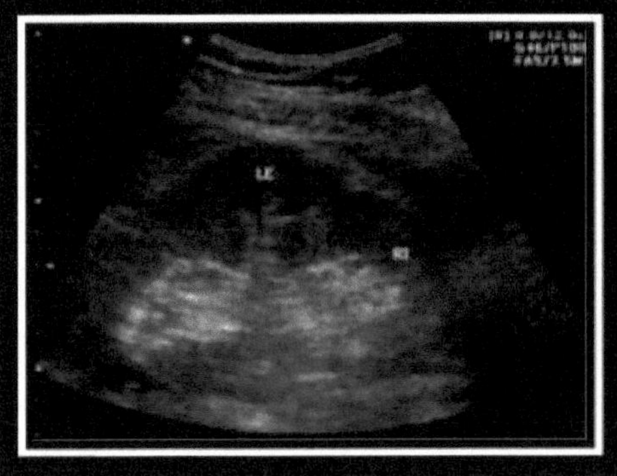

Ectopic rhinon
Ectopy is usually low and associated with renal malrotation.
Horseshoe rhinon

The kidneys are joined (at their lower pole) by a fibrous band or by renal parenchyma with their upper poles more lateral than their lower poles.
There is usually some degree of ectopia, and it can often be associated with hydronephrosis and cholelithiasis.

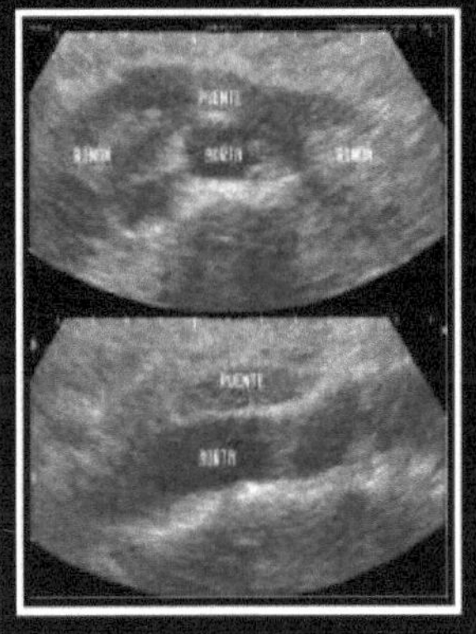

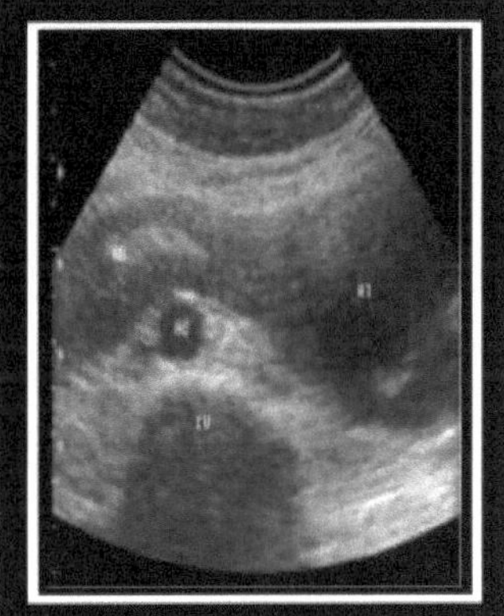

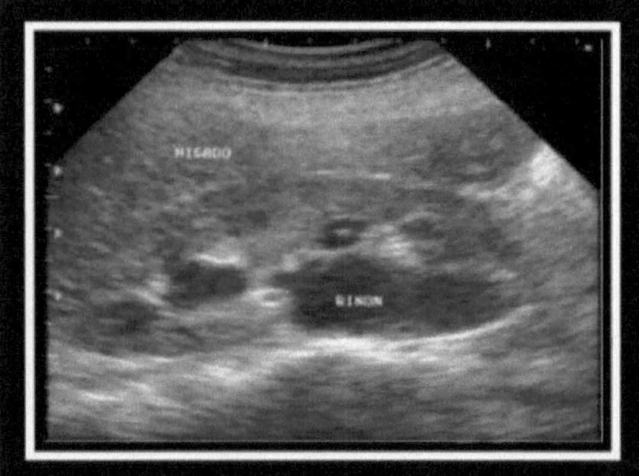

In this case the pelvis extends from the renal sinus towards the hilar fat. On ultrasound the pelvis is the only dilated part of the excretory system.
DUPLICATION OF THE COLLECTING SYSTEM
It may be an incomplete (bifid pelvis) or complete kidney with double collecting system, with bifid or double ureter. The ultrasound shows a large kidney with two echogenic renal sinuses separated by cortical tissue.

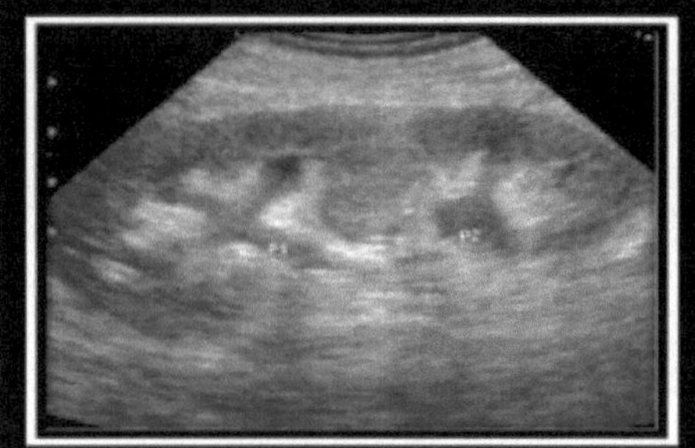

Benign neoplasm

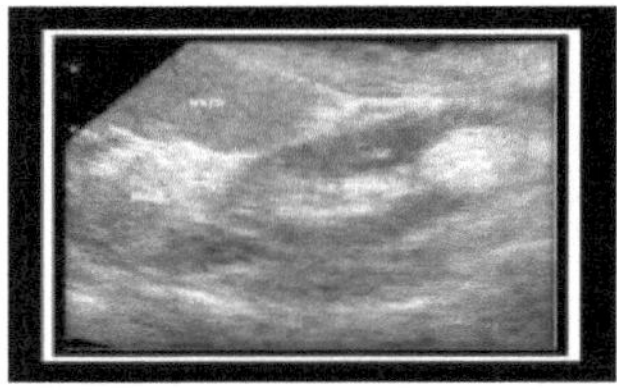

Mielolipoma

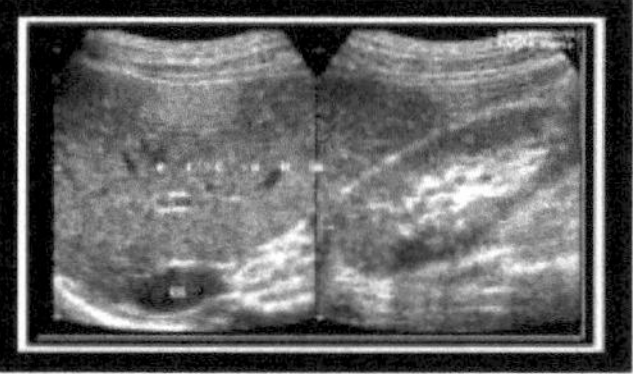

Adenoma cortical

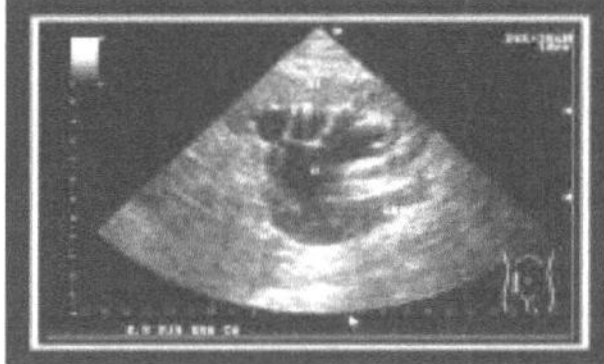

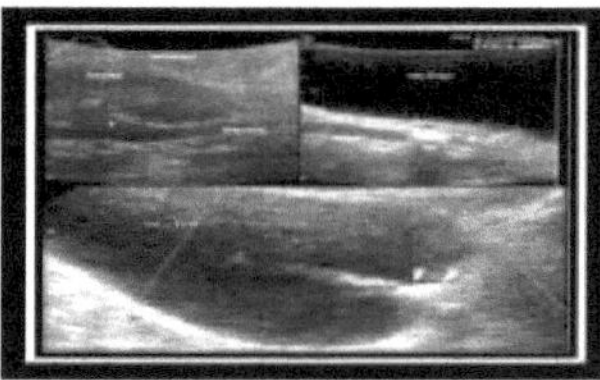

Litiasis ureteral

Myelolipoma Cortical adenoma
Ureteral lithiasis

Chapter 7

Ultrasound of the Supra Renal Glands

1 Malignant diseases to rule out metastases.
2 Addison's disease.
3 Cushing's disease and syndrome.
4 Abdominal tumour in a paediatric patient.
5 Virilism.
6 Sexual precocity.
7 Ambiguous genitalia.
8 Paroxysmal arterial hypertension.

Normal anatomy of GSRs.

The GSRs, surrounded by fat, are located in the retroperitoneal space, at the level of the 11th or 12th rib outside the spine, in a triangular shape.

As for their size, it can be observed that they decrease in size from foetal age (140 mm long) to the child and in the adult they reach a size between 20 and 40 mm.

The outer portion secretes steroids (cortisol, aldosterone, androgen and oestrogen) while the inner portion secretes catecholamines (dopamine, epinephrine, norepinephrine).

Preparation and Technique.

The study of GSRs requires no prior preparation.

The right GSR is studied in the supine decubitus position by placing the transducer in the intercostal spaces at the mid-axillary line and using the abdomen as an acoustic window to see how it is positioned behind the IVC.

The left-sided GSR is studied somewhat posteriorly, using the spleen as an acoustic window.

Pathological alterations of GSRs.

1 Benign lesions.
- GSR cysts.
- Congenital hyperplasia.
- Hypoplasia or congenital absence.
- Infections, abscesses and haemorrhages.
- Myelolipoma.
- Cortical adenoma.
2 Malignant lesions.
- Neuroblastoma.
- Adrenocortical carcinoma.
- Lymphomas.
- Metastasis.
- Pheochromocytoma.

Malignant neoplasms

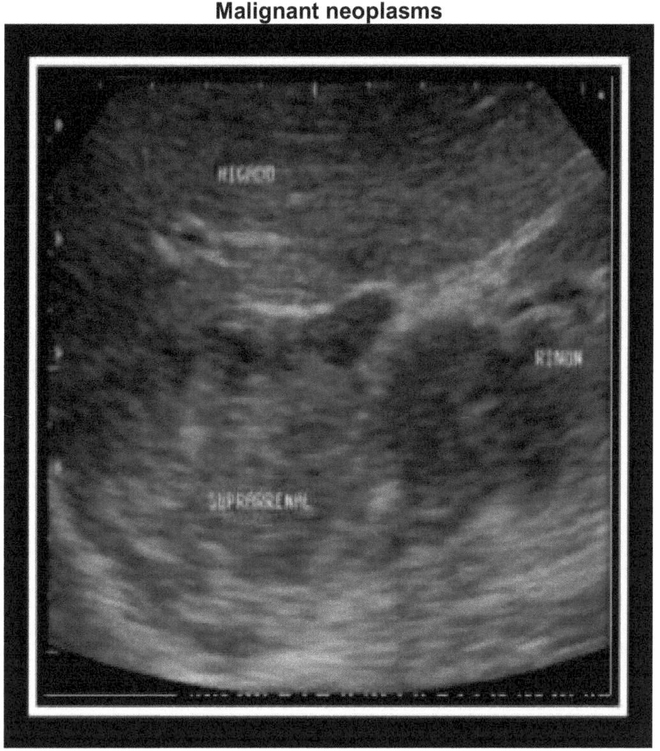

Chapter 8

Ultrasound of the Bladder, Prostate and Seminal Bladder.

Indications for Bladder US.
1. Haematuria.
2. Repeated urinary sepsis.
3. Difficulty in urination (dysuria).
4. Incontinence or urinary retention.
5. Pelvic tumour.
6. Pelvic trauma.
7. Disorders of the upper urinary tract which may have repercussions or origin in the bladder.

Approaches for the US study of the bladder.
- ❖ Suprapubic abdominal route.
- ❖ Transrectal route.
- ❖ Transvesical route.

Preparation and Technique.
(Via abdominal suprapubic).
- ❖ Bladder repletion (oral, intravenous or catheterised).
- ❖ Patient lying supine decubitus.
- ❖ 3.5 MHz transducer for adults and 5 MHz for children and very thin adults. The transducers can be linear or sectorial, preferably the latter because of their large scanning radius.
- ❖ Longitudinal, transversal and oblique cuts should be made from the pubic symphysis to the umbilicus, making movements in different directions for a complete exploration of the walls.
- ❖ Inspection of the upper urinary tract.

Functional study of the bladder.
Repletion and post micturition examination.
In the post-micturition phase, the existence of residual urine is evaluated by measuring the residual volume, using the largest transverse diameter, the height between the neck and the cup, the distance between the bottom and the cup; by multiplying these parameters we will obtain a fairly approximate value of the residual volume.

It is useful in the diagnosis of active vesico-ureteral reflux (in the voiding phase), in the study of neurogenic bladder and in outflow obstruction.

It also helps us to clarify diagnostic doubts with conditions in adjacent organs (e.g. giant ovarian cyst or prostatic alterations).

Normal Bladder Anatomy.
It appears as an anecogenic area located in the pelvis, symmetrical, with smooth and uniform walls. The thickness of the distended bladder is less than 4 mm. The emptying volume of the bladder is obtained by multiplying the transverse diameter by the longitudinal diameter by the anteroposterior diameter by the constant 0.52 and the result is expressed in ml.

Vol = DT x DL x DAP x 0.52 (ml).

Pathological alterations of the bladder.
It should be noted:
- Variations in wall thickness and the presence of trabeculations.
- Wall asymmetry.
- Hypoechogenic bladder masses (diverticula and ureteroceles).
- Solid masses in the bladder or towards the floor of the bladder.

<u>**Pathological alterations of the bladder.**</u>
<u>**(Generalised wall thickening).**</u>
1　In the male it is almost always an expression of distal prostatic or neck obstruction. It is frequently associated with diverticula.
2　Severe chronic cystitis. The inner wall of the bladder thickens and becomes regular.
3　Parasitism. Calcifications may be seen.
4　Bladder with highly trabeculated walls in the young child. Valva of posterior urethra.
5　Trabeculated walled bladder associated with neurogenic bladder.
<u>**Pathological alterations of the bladder.**</u>
<u>**(Localised wall thickening).**</u>
1　Bladder folds due to bladder not well distended (repeat the examination with a full bladder).
2　Sessile or pedunculated tumour, single or multiple.
3　Parasitic granulomatous infection.
4　Traumatic haematoma.
D.D:- Single or multiple neoplasia, with localised wall thickening, sometimes with wall infiltration and sometimes calcified.
-　Polyps. They are movable and their stalk can be seen.
-　Granuloma (TB). The bladder is small, with multiloculated thickening.
-　Trauma: The presence of blood in the vicinity should be investigated.
-　Coaguli: They offer a US image very similar to T.
<u>**Pathological alterations of the bladder.**</u>
<u>**(Intravesical masses).**</u>
- Masses attached to the wall:
1　Polyps. They are mobilised by a long pedicle.
2　Adherent calculus. The examination should be performed in different positions to try to mobilise it. There is SA.
3　Ureterocele. Located near the meatus and varying in shape and size, anomaKas or associated complications must be ruled out.
- Intravesical mobile masses:
1　Lithiasis: when they are small or medium-sized, they can be mobilised, but not when they occupy a large part of the bladder or are inside a diverticulum.
2　Foreign body. Catheters or foreign body.
3　Blood clots.
4　Air: from outside or from intestinal ffstula.
<u>**Pathological alterations of the bladder.**</u>
<u>**(Megaveiiga).**</u>
1　Prostatic enlargement.
2　Urethral stricture in men.
3　Urethral lithiasis in men.
4　Urethritis in women.
5　Neurogenic bladder.
6　Ureteral valves in the newborn.
7　Cystocele in some patients.
<u>**Pathological alterations of the bladder.**</u>
<u>**(Small bladder).**</u>
1　Recurrent cystitis. TB, parasitosis.
2　Infiltrating neoplasia.
3　RGT or surgery for neoplasms.

<u>**Pathological alterations of neighbouring organs.**</u>
1   Prostatic hyperplasia raises the bladder floor and causes a fighting bladder.
2   Uterine fibroids cause compression of the bladder wall.
3   Malignant tumours of the ovary, uterus, prostate, seminal vesicles and rectum may compress or invade the bladder.
4   Inflammatory, lymphomatous or metastatic adenomegalies deform the bladder contour by compression.
5   Intrapelvic haematomas compress the bladder wall.
<u>**Traumatic bladder injuries.**</u>
1   It is caused by direct trauma to the distended bladder, pelvic fracture or bladder instrumentation accident.
2   The rupture may be intraperitoneal or retroperitoneal.
3   If it is intraperitonial we can observe free fluid (urine) in the peritoneal cavity, in the parietocolic spaces or in other sites of decline.
4   If the rupture is extraperitoneal, the Kquido decoles the pelvic space and displaces the bladder upwards or sideways.
5   Most frequently, the bladder is empty and we are unable to achieve its repletion, observing free fluid in the pelvic space.

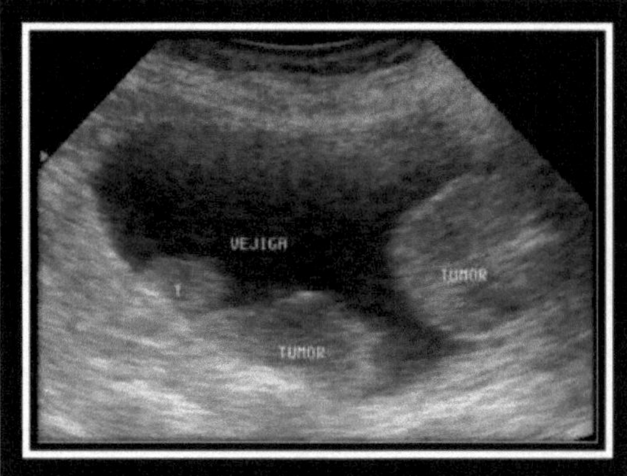

Bladder Tumour

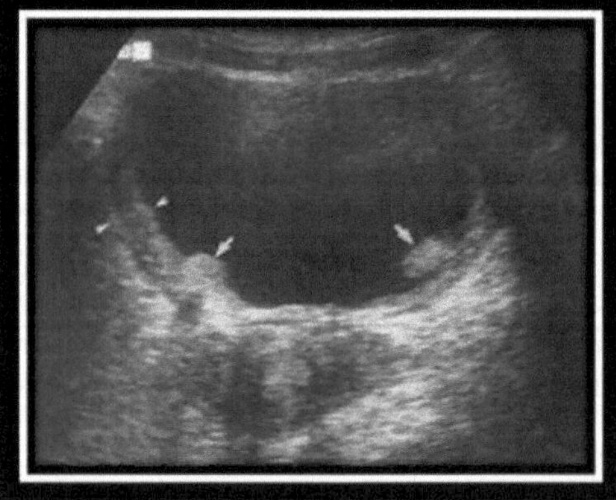

Infectious cystitis

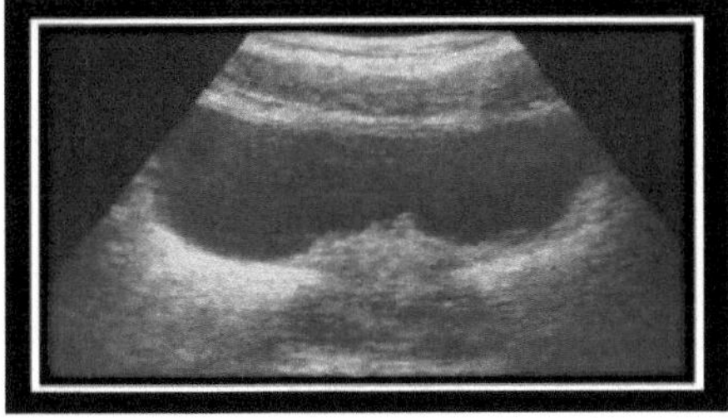

Masa de implantación mucosa con invasión focal de próstata

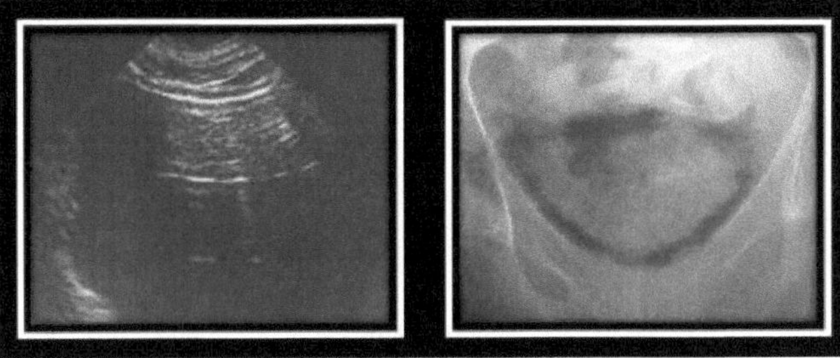

Cistitis enfisematosa

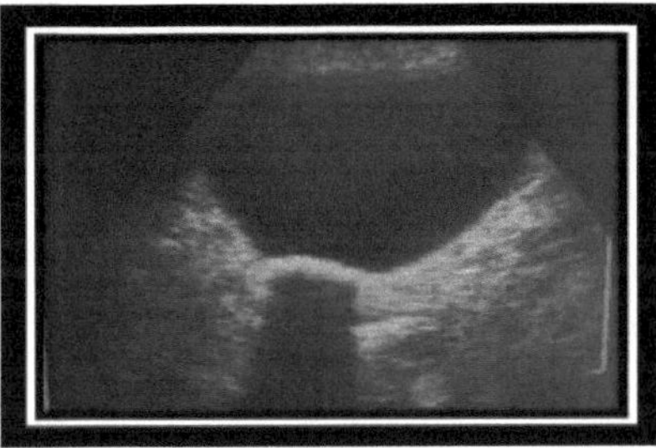

Cálculo vesical

Mucosal implantation mass with focal prostate invasion
Emphysematous cystitis
Bladder stones

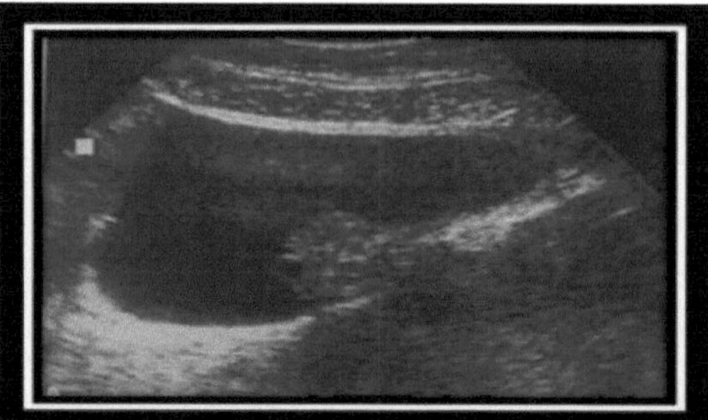

Bladder endometriosis

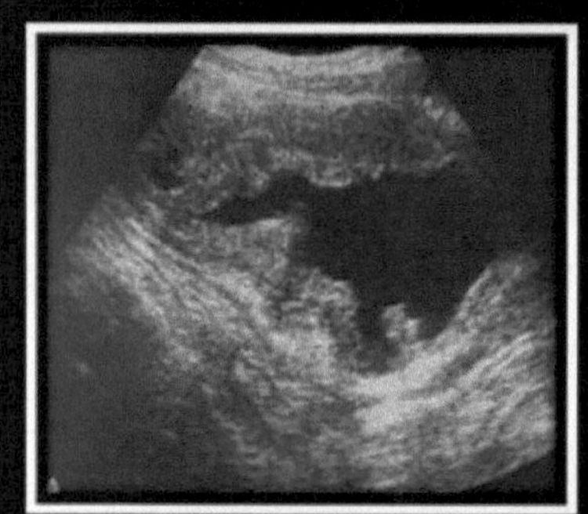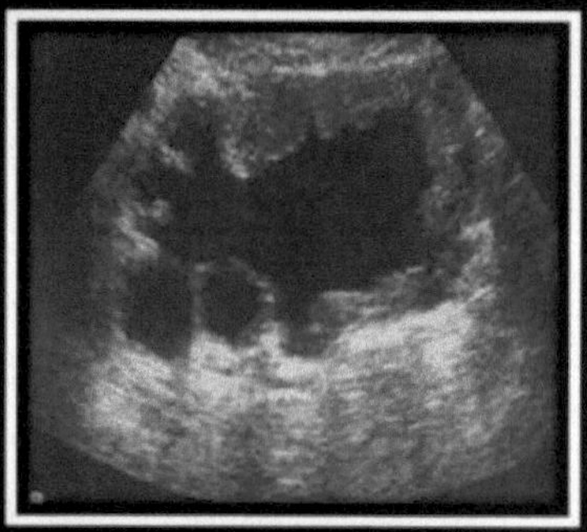

Thickening of the trabeculae of the bladder walls.

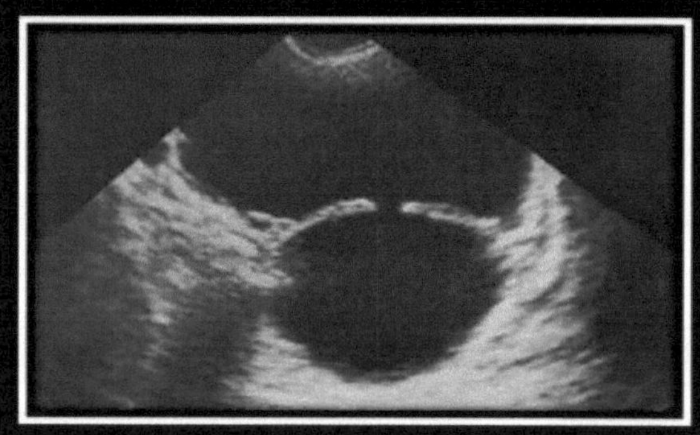

Bladder diverticulum

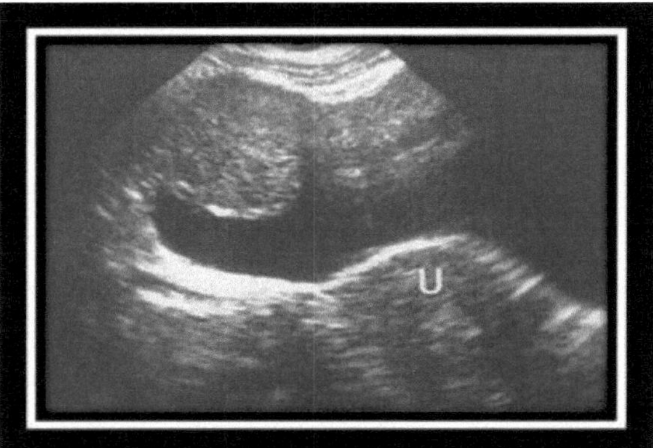

Bladder tumour

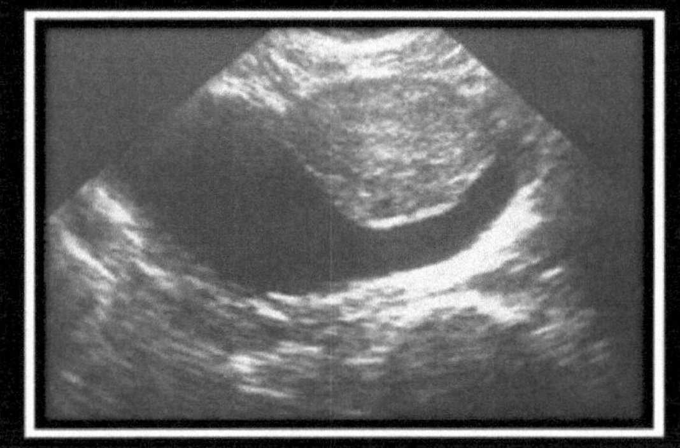

Bladder tumour

Chapter 9

Prostate Ultrasound.

Indications for prostate US.
1 Difficulty in urination (dysuria).
2 Urinary sepsis.
3 Urinary retention.
4 Haematuria.
5 Perineal pain.
6 Manifestations in other organs or systemic manifestations that raise suspicion of prostatic neoplasia.
7 In screening for prostatic carcinoma.

Approach routes for the US study of the prostate.
* Via suprapubica.
* Transrectal route.

Suprapubic abdominal route.
Examination with a full bladder, avoiding bladder overdistention.
Use 3.5 and 5 MHz transducers.
Perform coronal, longitudinal and oblique cuts.

Longitudinal section: the prostate is partially hidden by the symphysis pubis, it is shaped like a walnut.

Coronal section: its shape is rounded or quadrangular. It should be performed by placing the transducer at an angle between 15° and 30° in the caudal direction.

Anatomy of the Prostate.
It is located in the lesser pelvis below the bladder and above the urogenital diaphragm, in the mid-abdominal line, behind the pubic symphysis.

It contains the urethra, which extends from the base to the apex, centrally located cephalo-caudally and slightly anterior to the midline.

Weighs approximately 20gs.

In axial section it is walnut-shaped and in longitudinal section it is pyramidal in appearance. The normal prostate weighs approximately 20 grams. The increase in its volume is classified into 4 grades:

Grade I: 20 to 30 grams
Grade II: 30 to 50 grams
Grade III: 50 to 85 grams
Grade IV: more than 85 grams

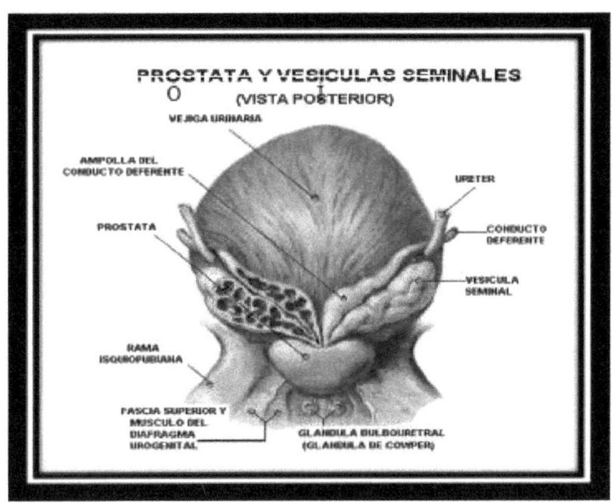

PROSTATA Y VESÍCULAS SEMINALES
(VISTA POSTERIOR)
VEJIGA URINARIA
AMPOLLA DEL CONDUCTO DEFERENTE
URETER
PROSTATA
CONDUCTO DEFERENTE
VESÍCULA SEMINAL
RAMA ISQUIOPUBIANA
FASCIA SUPERIOR Y MÚSCULO DEL DIAFRAGMA UROGENITAL
GLÁNDULA BULBOURETRAL (GLÁNDULA DE COWPER)

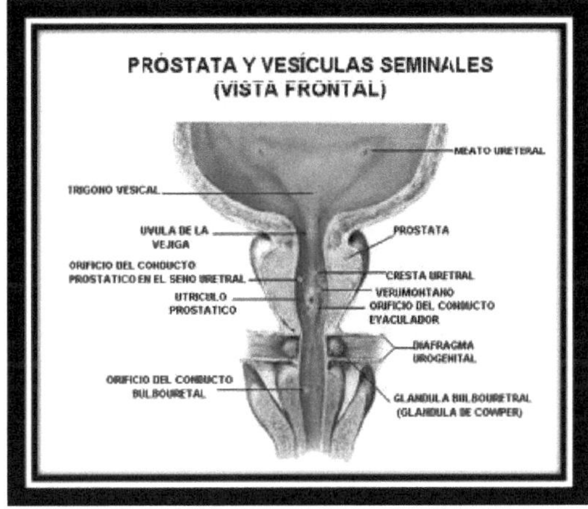

PRÓSTATA Y VESÍCULAS SEMINALES
(VISTA FRONTAL)
MEATO URETERAL
TRÍGONO VESICAL
ÚVULA DE LA VEJIGA
PRÓSTATA
ORIFICIO DEL CONDUCTO PROSTÁTICO EN EL SENO URETRAL
CRESTA URETRAL
ÚTRICULO PROSTÁTICO
VERUMONTANO
ORIFICIO DEL CONDUCTO EYACULADOR
DIAFRAGMA UROGENITAL
ORIFICIO DEL CONDUCTO BULBOURETRAL
GLÁNDULA BULBOURETRAL (GLÁNDULA DE COWPER)

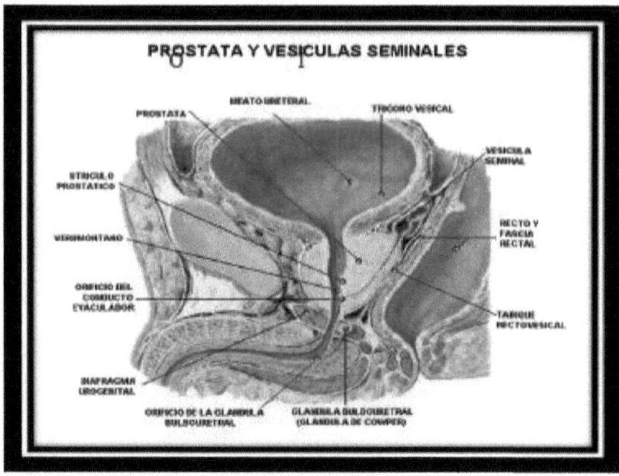

<u>Ultrasonographic appearance of the prostate.</u>

The normal gland is echogenic in appearance, homogeneous; outlined by a hyperechoic rim representing capsular echogram corresponding to periprostatic fat.

It has a peripheral zone (70%) where more than 25% of carcinomas are located. A pre-prostatic region (urethral segment), the exclusive site of benign hyperplasia.

<u>Zonal Anatomical Model Mc Neil</u>

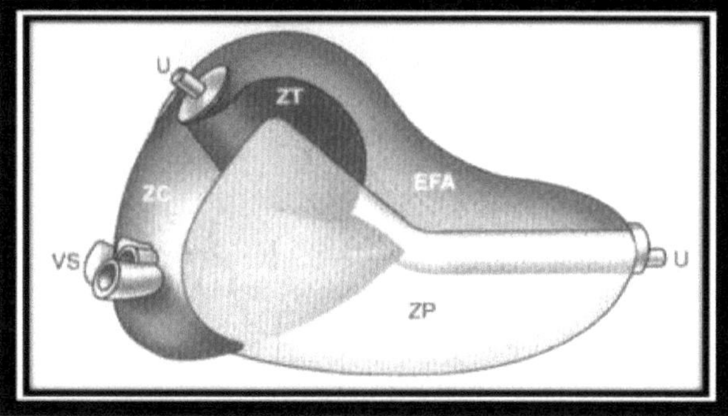

<u>Zt: transition zone, ZP: peripheral zone, ZC: central zone, EFA: anterior fibromu scular stromal, U: urethra, VS: seminal vesicles.</u>

Proximal urethra
Uretra proximal

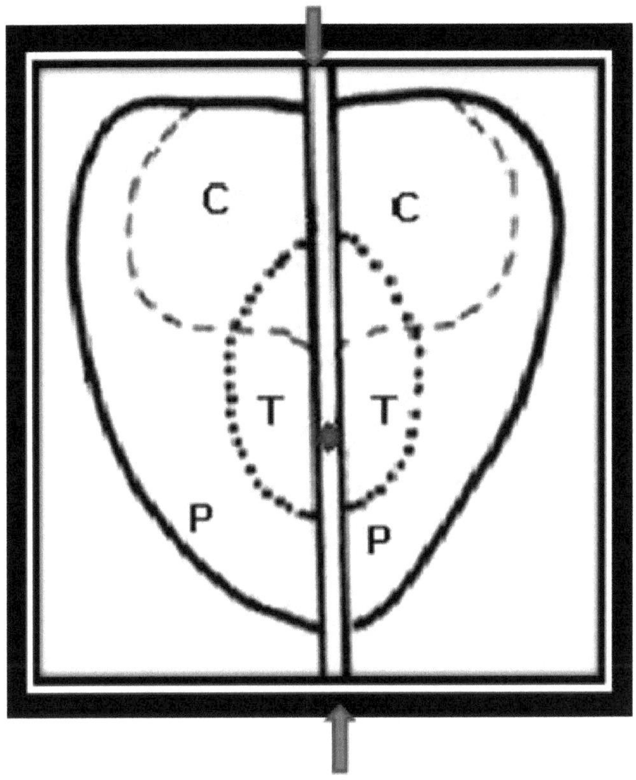
C
C
T
T
P
P

Uretra distal
Distal urethra

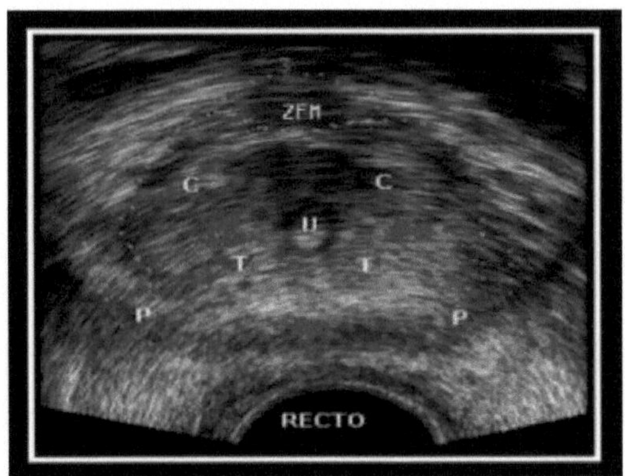

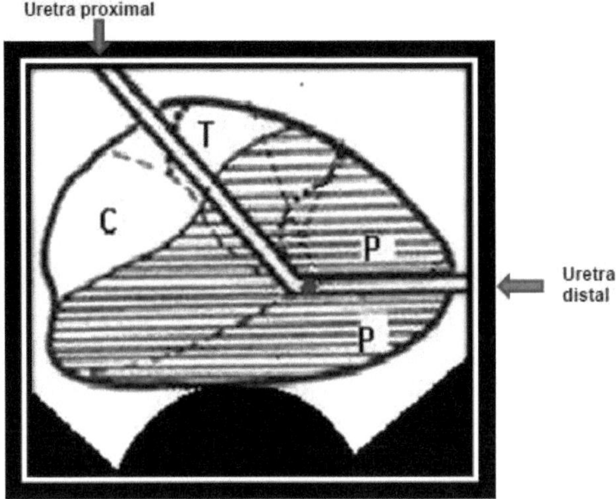

Proximal urethra
Distal urethra

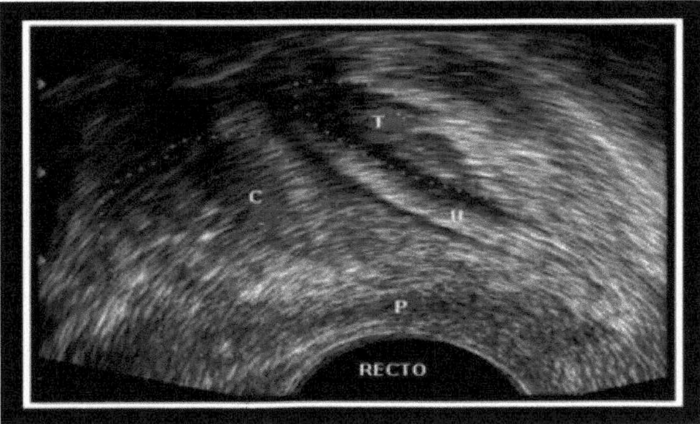

Pathological alterations of the prostate.
(Prostatitis).

Acute:
- Generally the appearance of the gland is normal.
- May appear slightly enlarged and/or hypoechoic. chronic:
- Non-homogeneous ultrasonographic image of echogenic predominance, with or without calcifications.
- Well-defined outline, may be irregular.
- The volume of the gland is usually increased, although it may also appear decreased.
- Difficult to differentiate from diffuse carcinoma.

Pathological alterations of the prostate.
(Hyperplasia).

- Volume increase.
- Well-defined, generally regular contours.
- Homogeneous texture.

Pathological alterations of the prostate.
(Carcinoma).

Initial stage.
- Nodular form. may occur anywhere on the gland, but predominate at the vertex (caudal end).
Echogenic or hypoechoic in appearance.
- Diffuse form. inhomogeneity of acoustic distribution (complex appearance), ill-defined Kmite, partially or completely occupying the gland.
The prostatic contour may be irregular or ill-defined.
The difference with chronic prostatitis is difficult.

Advanced stage.

The ultrasonographic image of the gland is very complex.

Edges are not defined.

Regional lymph node metastases and bladder floor invasion are common.

Uni or bilateral hydronephrosis due to bladder trigone seizure.

Distant metastases.

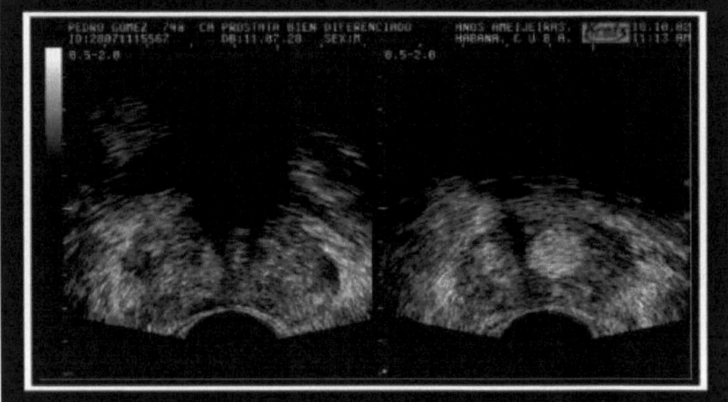

Carcinoma of the prostate (transrectal route)

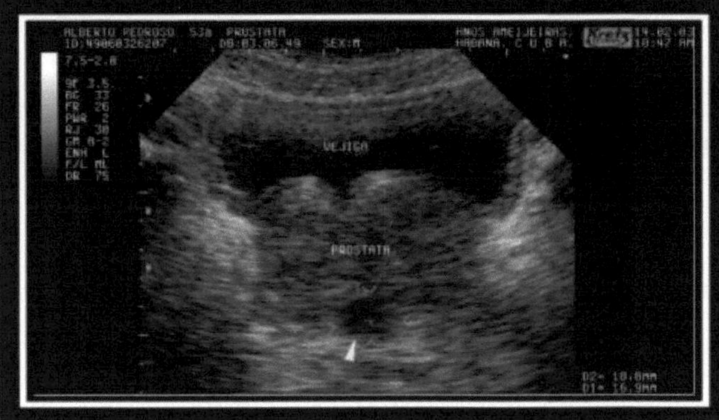

Carcinoma of the prostate (Via suprapubic)

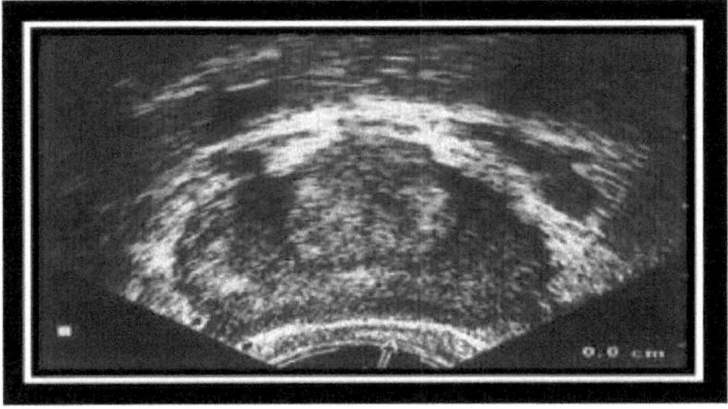

Hiperplasia próstática (Vía transrectal)

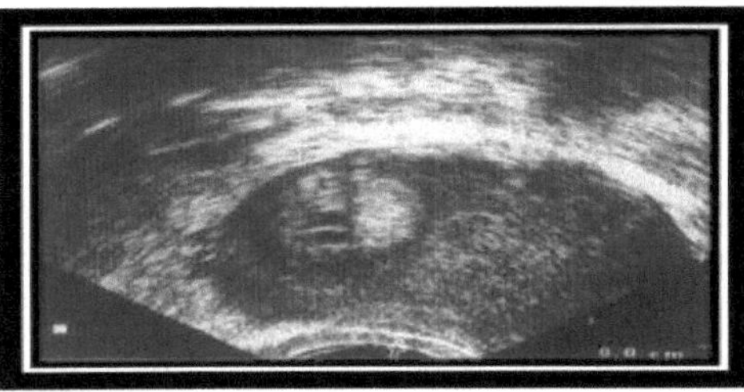

Formación nodular hiperecoica con áreas quísticas   (Vía transrectal)

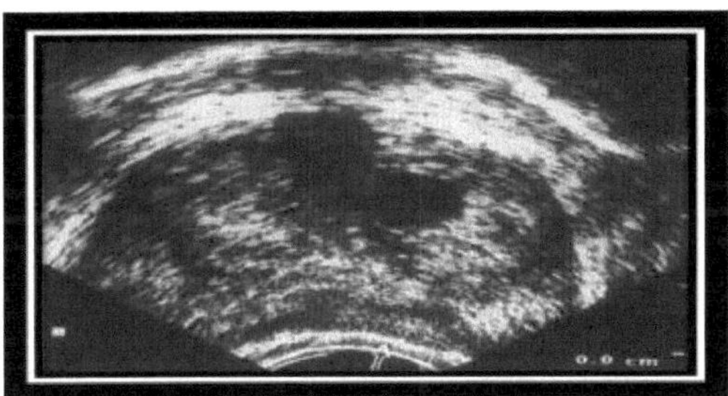

Prostatic hyperplasia (Transrectal route)
Hyperechoic nodular formation with cystic areas (Transrectal route)

ANECHOIC FORMATION IN LEFT CENTRAL AREA IN RELATION TO RETENTION CYST

Chapter 10

Ultrasound of the Seminal Vesicles.

Indications for Seminal Vesicle US.

1   Infertility under study.
2   Azoospermia.
3   Hemospermia.
4   Dilatations of the seminal vesicles.
5   Suspicion of cysts.
6   Suspected prostatic tumours with infiltration of seminal vesicles.

Examination technique and ultrasonographic anatomy.

Coronal sections are made in the mid-abdominal line at the infra-umbilical level, with a caudal angulation of the transducer of 15° to 20° , the prostate is located and sections are made at 0.5 cm intervals above its upper edge until both vesfcules appear.

Generally symmetrical and incurved.

Shape variable: rounded, elongated, often rectangular.

Its largest diameter is the transverse.

Anatomy

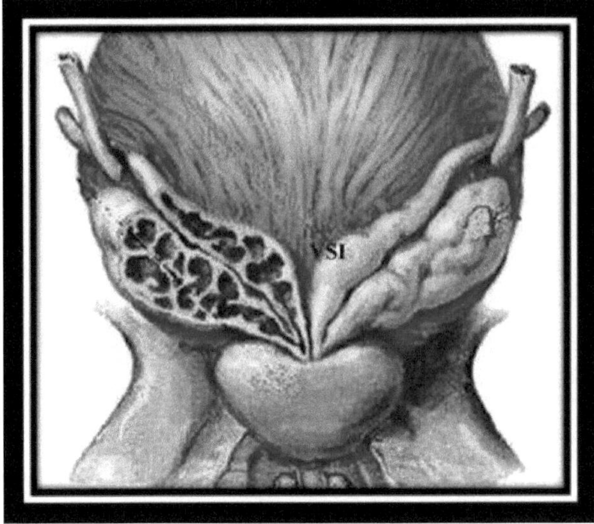

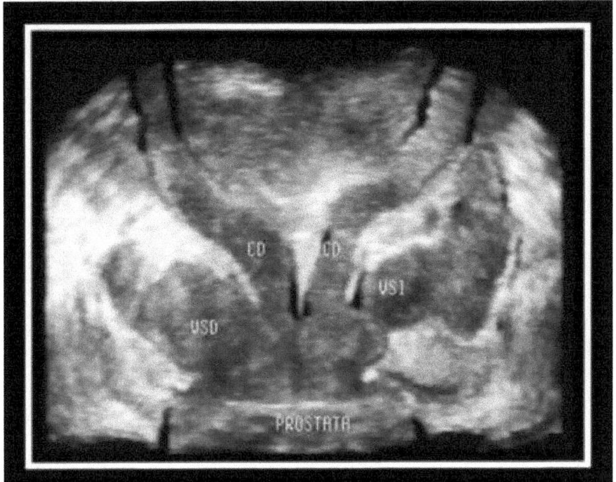

Ecograffa 3D

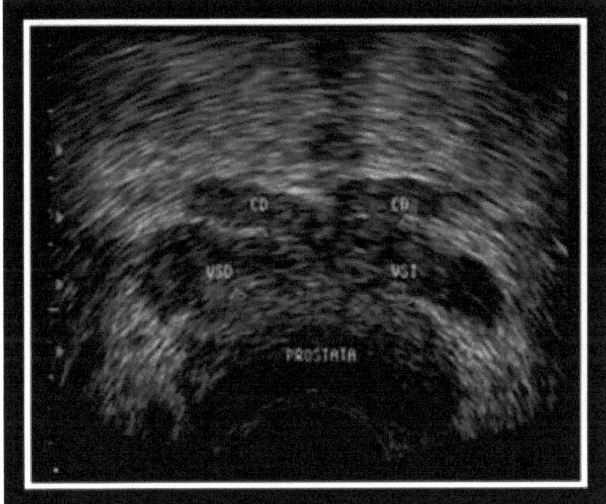

2D Ultrasound

<u>**Most frequent pathological alterations.**</u>
- Congenital anomaKas. Agenesis
Hypoplasia.
- Cysts.
- Tumours.

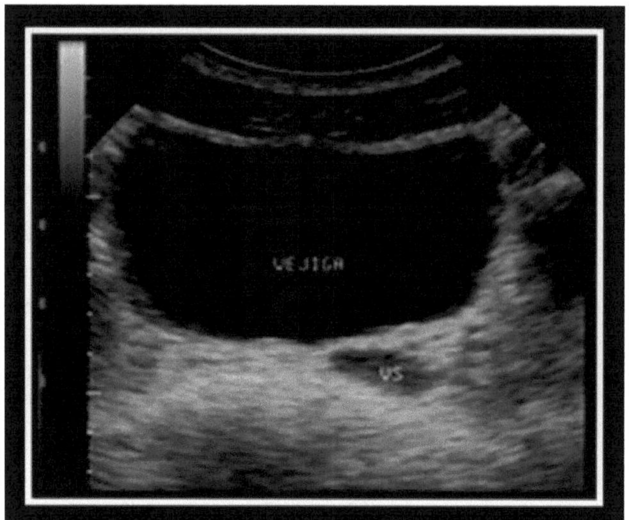

Agenesis of the right seminal vesicle

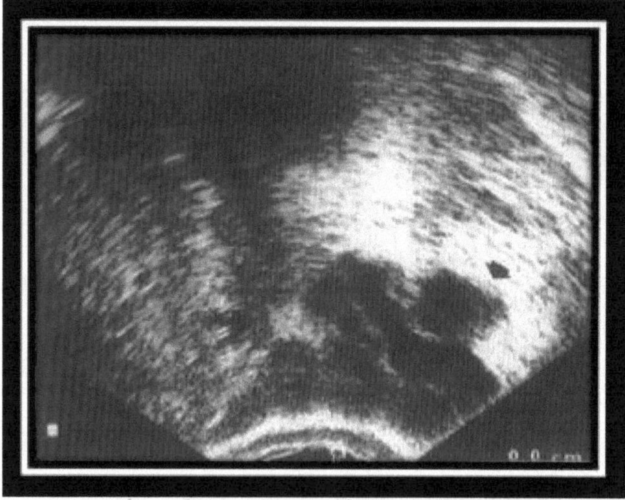

Dilatación quística de la vesícula seminal derecha.
Cystic dilatation of the right seminal vesicle.

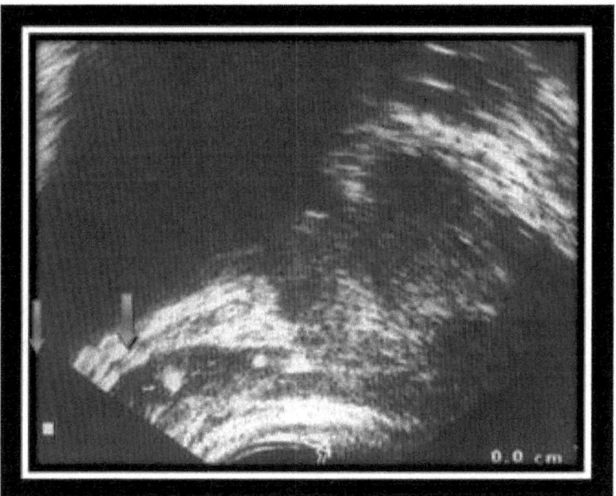

Hyperechoic areas inside the right seminal vesicle

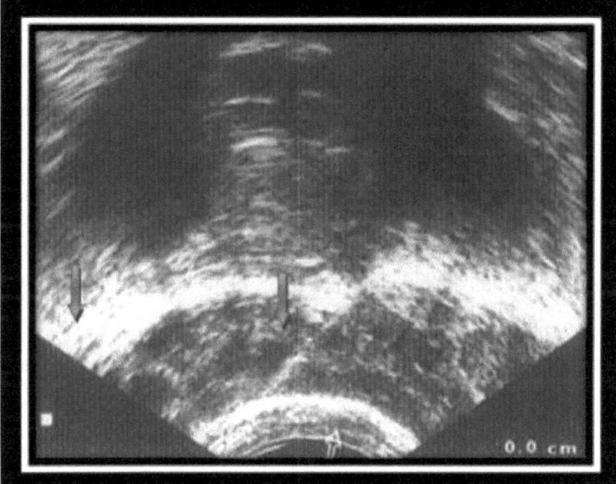

Dilatation of both seminal vesicles.

Chapter 11

Ultrasound of the Peritoneal Cavity and GIT.

Indications for US of the peritoneal cavity and GIT.

- Adults:

1   Localised abdominal pain.
2   Abdominal mass.
3   Suspected ascites or peritonitis.
4   Suspected appendicitis.

- Children:

1   Suspected hypertrophic pyloric stenosis.
2   Suspicion of intestinal intussusception.

Preparation and Technique.

Fasting patient in decubitus supine position with transducers ranging from 3.5 MHz to 7 MHz. Longitudinal, transverse and oblique slices should be made of the whole abdomen. The technique of phonographic palpation is very useful.

Normal anatomy of the GIT.

Oesophagus: the abdominal portion of the oesophagus can be visualised by making longitudinal cuts parallel to the Ao or coronal cuts behind the left hepatic lobe.

Stomach: when empty, the fundus is star-shaped, while the body can be seen in front of the pancreas in cross-sections. Ingestion of Kquido can make it easier and clearer to visualise.

Small and large intestine: Its appearance varies depending on its contents and above all on the amount of liquid, gas and faeces. Peristalsis and mobile echoes can be seen inside. The intestinal wall shows two layers of echoes: an external or muscular hypoechogenic layer and an internal or mucosal layer in contact with the intestinal contents, which appears hyperechogenic. The intestinal gas is hyperechogenic and produces reverberation phenomena as well as posterior SA.

Pathological alterations of the PC and GIT.
(Hypertrophic pyloric stenosis).

In case of clinical suspicion, US can confirm the diagnosis by showing a hypoechogenic area no larger than 4 cm, which corresponds to muscular hypertrophy, associated with gastric stasis and hyperperistalsis. In CL at the level of the pylorus, the lesion is seen to be more than 2 cm long.

Pathological alterations of the PC and GIT.
(Appendicitis).

The examination should be performed with gentle manoeuvres and phonographic palpation technique.

In CC the inflamed appendix appears as a fixed circular structure with a hypoechogenic lumen surrounded by a hyperechogenic area of oedema. It is not uncommon to see some bowel loops neighbouring the appendix.

In CS the appendix takes a tubular shape. If perforation has occurred, an irregularly contoured or complex echolucent area may be seen adjacent to the appendix and extending into the pelvic cavity.

Pathological alterations of the PC and GIT.
(Invagination).

In the presence of clinical suspicion in U:S, the invaginated loop may be visualised, especially on CT scans showing a series of concentric rings with a hypoechogenic ring greater than 8 mm thick.

In these cases, US can not only be used for diagnosis, but can also be used as a guide to perform the appropriate manoeuvres to de-vaginate the loops.

Pathological alterations of the PC and GIT.
(Parasitosis).
Ascaris lumbricoides: They appear as concentric rings within the lumen of the intestinal loops, and mobility can often be visualised in them. If we make the patient ingest water, when it reaches the site occupied by the Ascaris lumbricoides, the image becomes clearer.
Pathological alterations of the PC and GIT.
(Ascites).
US is of great value in the identification of free fluid in the PC, this will be seen as an anechogenic image that conforms to the anatomical structures or if it is a tension ascites we can see displacement of the anatomical structures with all or almost all their walls and contours well defined by the window provided by the asdtic fluid.
The hypogastrium and Morrison's space are the first places where asdic content is evident (regions of decline).
Pathological alterations of the PC and GIT.
(Intestinal masses).
The presence of a solid mass should rule out an inflammatory (abscess) or neoplastic process. Tumours of the bowel have a reniform appearance, with poorly defined borders. Neighbouring adenopaUas and possible hepatic metastases should be looked for as indirect signs.
Pathological alterations of the PC and GIT.
(Extraintestinal masses).
They are usually due to lymphoma and present as hypoechogenic masses. Other causes may be retroperitoneal sarcomas which cause larger masses with variable echogenicity and frequent central necrosis.
Pathological alterations of the PC and GIT.
(Complex masses).
They produce an ill-defined irregular area.
Possible causes include:
-   Appendicular abscess.
-   Diverticulitis with perforation.
-   Amebiasis with perforation.
-   Perforated neoplasia.
-   Intestinal TB.
Pathological alterations of the PC and GIT (haematomas).
They produce a cystic or complex mass, very similar to an abscess, with echogenic material inside and sometimes loculated.
Pathological alterations of the PC and GIT.
(Masses filled with liquid).
-   Intestinal duplicity: may have internal echoes from waste material or septa.
-   Mesenteric cyst: may have septa.
-   Parasitic cyst: echogenic images can sometimes be seen inside the cyst.
-   Intestinal ischaemia: This is a localised thickened area in the bowel wall without peristalsis.
Pathological alterations of the PC and GIT.
(AIDS infection).
US is very useful especially in patients with a febrile syndrome to rule out possible abscesses or adenopaUas. In addition, the liver, spleen, kidneys, pelvis and pelvis should be explored, as well as careful emphasis on subphrenic regions, and the pericave, periaortic and pelvic adenopaUas should be localised.
Ascites

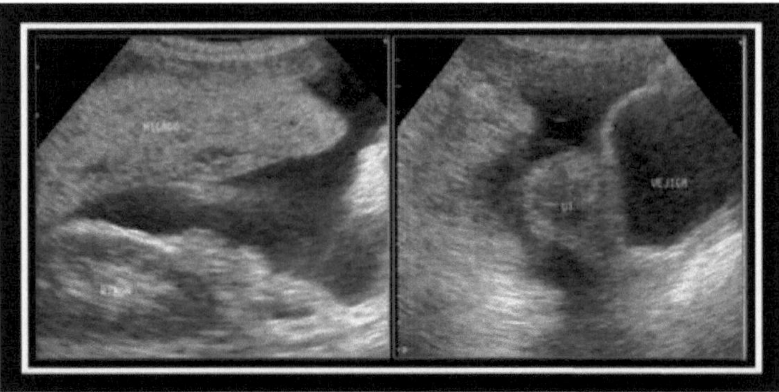

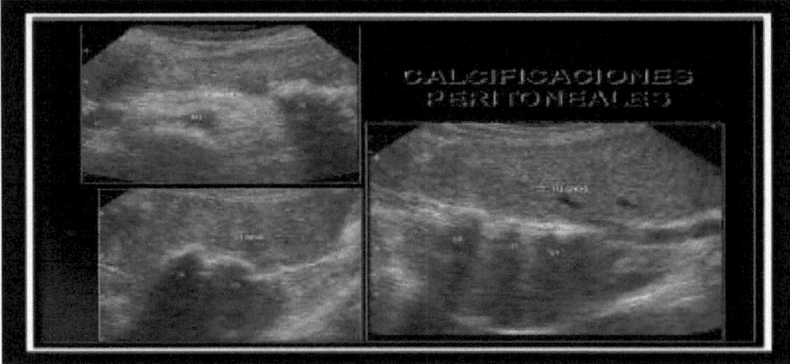
CALCIFICACIONES
PERITONEALES

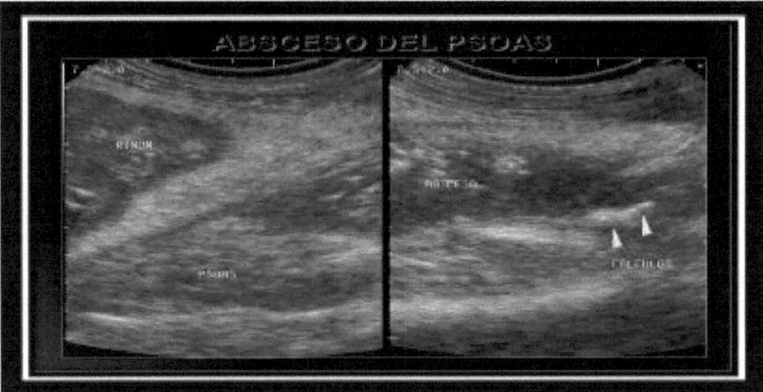
ABSCESO DEL PSOAS

Chapter 12

Gynaecological Ultrasound.

Indications for gynaecological US.

1   Pelvic pain, including dysmenorrhoea.
2   Pelvic mass.
3   Abnormal vaginal bleeding.
4   Abnormal vaginal discharge.
5   Amenorrhoea.
6   Confirm the existence and location of an IUD.
7   Infertility.
8   Low urinary symptoms.
9   Diffuse abdominal pain.
10 Follicular monitoring.

Preparation and Technique.

The examination should be performed with a full bladder, decubitus supine with transducers between 3.5 and 5 MHz. Longitudinal and parasagittal midline and parasagittal cuts are made from the pubis to the umbilicus and then transversal cuts. For the study of the ovaries, oblique cuts of 30 to 40 degrees are necessary.

Transvaginal US. A special transducer is required and the test is performed with the bladder empty.

Normal gynaecological US anatomy.

In a CS, the vagina is identified behind and below the bladder, with its hypoechogenic walls and the vaginal mucosa inside, which is more echogenic. Above, the uterus is seen, with its hypoechogenic peripheral muscular layer and the thin endometrium, whose echogenicity increases in the premenstrual phase.

The normal postpubertal uterus measures 4.5 - 9.0 cm in length by 1.5 - 3 cm AP and 4.5 - 5.5 cm in transverse diameter.

In girls before puberty the uterus is smaller than the neck, which is reversed during adolescence.

Normal gynaecological US anatomy.

CT scans should be done with posterior and downward angulation, trying to identify the vagina, the rectum and the lower portion of the bladder, then the ligaments on both sides of the mid lhea and the ovaries from the bottom up.

It should be remembered that after each pregnancy the uterus increases in size and its body becomes more rounded while in the post menopausal woman the uterus decreases in size and becomes more homogeneous and the endometrial cavity is not visible. The same is true of the ovaries.

The normal uterus may not be in the middle of the uterus and may also rotate about its own major axis or be angulated.

The normal pattern of the endometrium varies with the menstrual cycle, appearing thin and hypoechogenic at the beginning of the cycle, hyperechogenic in mid-cycle surrounded by a hypoechogenic halo, and during menstruation the endometrial cavity thickens and becomes hyperechogenic.

The IUD placed in the endometrial cavity is visualised as an echogenic structure with SA.

The ovaries outside the uterus appear as ovoid structures, less homogeneous than the uterus but with the same echogenicity.

Sometimes they are situated in a cul-de-sac or very high above the uterus.

When the ovary is not well identified, it is advisable to place the patient in an oblique position and study the ovary opposite the transducer using the acoustic window offered by the bladder, as well as adjusting the gains of the equipment appropriately.

Ovarian foKculi appear as anecogenic spaces in or around the ovarian surface and can measure up to 5 cm, which makes it necessary to perform evolutive studies. These foKculi disappear during the menstrual cycle or can be resistant foKculi, sometimes they are made surgically or can be punctured.

It is not uncommon to find a small amount of fluid in the posterior fornix after ovulation or menstruation.

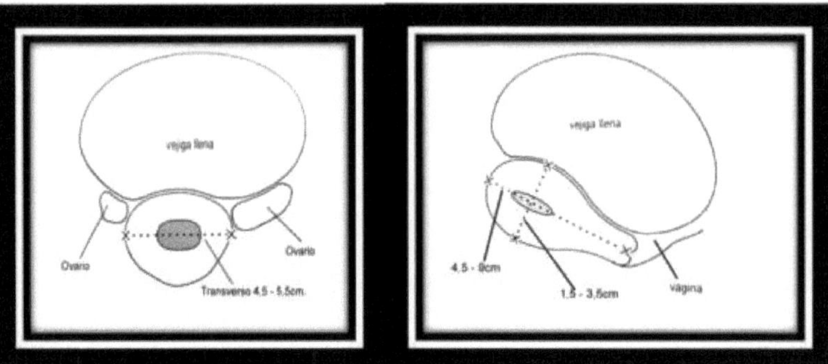

Physiological variations of the endometrium.

Postmenstrual period: No mucosa, the lhea de vacuidad is seen. Occasionally a physiological haematometra may be observed.

Proliferative phase: Hypoechoic mucosa surrounding the vacuity line.

Ovulatory phase: The pre-ovulatory corona appears.

Secretory phase: thick, hyperechogenic endometrium.

Normal endometrial thickness.

In premenopausal women:
- End of menses: 1 - 4 mm.
- Proliferative phase: 4 - 8 mm.
- Secretory phase: 12 - 16 mm.

In postmenopausal women: Up to 10 mm.

Pathological alterations of the uterus.
(Developmental AnomaKas).

1   Bicornuate uterus with two endometrial canals and two uterine fundi.
2   Double uterus with two endometrial canals and two cervical canals.
3   Imperforate hymen. There is accumulation of blood in the endometrium (haematometra) or in the vagina (haematocolpos) which makes it hypoechogenic. Sometimes it becomes infected and pus accumulates not only in the cavity (pyometra), but also in the fallopian tubes (piosalpin).

Lesions inside the Vagina.

1   Air in the vagina.
2   Urine.
3   Foreign bodies.
4   Haematocolpos in childhood.
5   Tumours (rare).
6   Gartner's duct cysts.

Cystic structures in the cervix.

1   Nabothian cysts.
2   Abortion in progress.
3   Cervical pregnancy.
4   Post-treatment liquid.
5   Necrotic cervical carcinoma.

Uterine enlargement.
1   Uterine fibroids.
2   Postpartum and multiparity period.
3   Hormonal stimulation.
4   Leiomyomatous involvement.
5   Endometrial carcinoma.
6   Obstructed uterus.

Pathological alterations of the uterus.
(Fibromas).
They present as nodular masses, almost always multiple, well-defined, homogeneous, peripherally located.

At the beginning they are hypoechogenic and with time they become hyperechogenic or with a mixed structure, due to necrosis or they may present calcifications.

Sometimes they are pedunculated and are mistaken for adnexal structures.

Pathological alterations of the uterus.
(Malignant tumours).
- Endometrial carcinoma.

Any postmenopausal woman with vaginal bleeding and an ultrasonographically thickened endometrium of more than 1 cm should be suspected of having endometrial carcinoma, even if it is not the main cause.

The endometrium becomes hyperplastic and hypoechogenic, and may extend into the myometrium, with distension of the cavity and the appearance of necrosis and cervical cancer. It is difficult to diagnose at first. It then causes thickening of the neck, with infiltration of neighbouring structures (bladder, vagina, rectum or peritoneum).

Increased endometrial thickness.
1   Normal secretory phase of the endometrium.
2   Endo and exogenous hormone stimulation.
3   Hyperplastic endometrium (cystic hyperplasia).
4   Polyps.
5   Endometrial carcinoma.
6   Endometritis.
7   Material inside the cavity.

Ovarian cycle.
1   Follicular phase.
2   Pre-ovulatory phase.
3   Ovulatory phase.
4   Lutemic phase.

Pathological alterations of the ovary.
(Cysts).
Most of them are follicles that do not rupture, are thin-walled, anecogenic.

Sometimes they are located behind the uterus or the bladder and when they are small they are difficult to visualise.

When very large, they grow into the abdomen and displace neighbouring structures. Sometimes they are complicated by internal echoes due to haemorrhages, nodules or septa. When the wall is thick, with a complex internal pattern, a malignant nature must be considered.

Dermoid cysts or teratomas present as solid or complex structures, with HS due to calcifications.

A cystic mass in the pelvis of a postmenopausal woman should raise suspicion of malignancy.

Simple adnexal cysts.
1   Functional ovarian cysts (FoKculous).

2   Paraovarian cysts.
3   ovarian cystic neoplasms (serous cystadenoma).
4   Peritoneal inclusion cysts (history of surgery or trauma).
5   Paraovarian cysts originate from the broad ligament.
6   They do not usually respond to hormonal changes.

<u>Pathological alterations of the ovaries.</u>
<u>(Complex adnexal mass).</u>

The causes outlined above.
1   Endometrioma.
2   tubo-ovarian abscess & hydrosalpinx.
3   Metastatic involvement of the ovary (GIT, breast and thyroid).
4   Primary ovarian neoplasia.
-    Germ cell tumour.
-    Epithelial tumours.
-    Stromal cell tumours.
5   Ectopic pregnancy.
6   Ovarian torsion.

<u>Pathological alterations of the ovaries.</u>
<u>(Ovarian tumours).</u>

1   Neoplasms of the superficial epithelium (70%).
-    Serous tumour.
-    Mucinous tumour.
-    Endometroid tumour.
-    Brener's tumour.
2   Neoplasms of the gonadal stroma.
3   Lipoid cell neoplasms.
4   Germ cell neoplasms (15%).
- Teratoma.
5   Mixed gonadal and germinal neoplasms.
6   Mesenchymal neoplasms.
7   Unclassified neoplasms.
8   Metastatic neoplasms (10%).

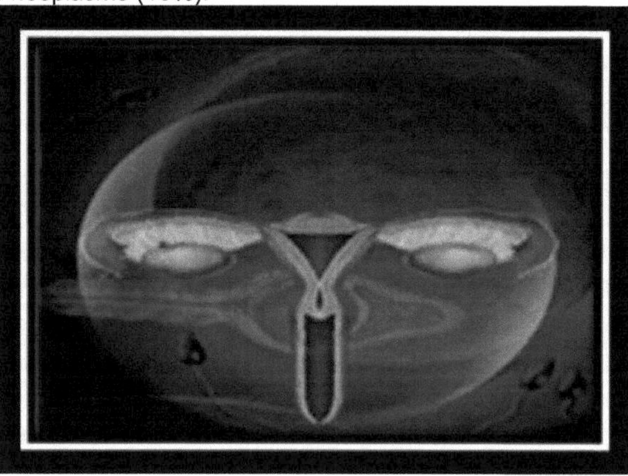

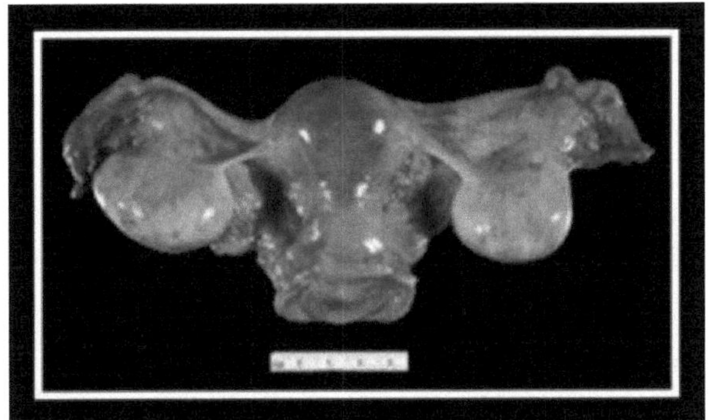

Most frequent anomalies

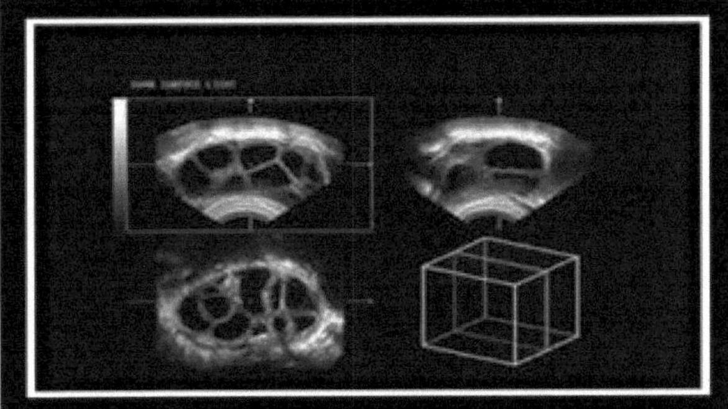

Polycystic Ovaries

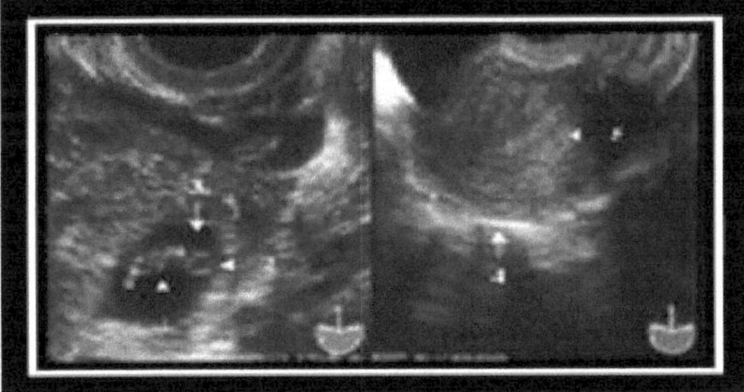

Transvaginal ultrasonographic image of unruptured ectopic pregnancy with embryo and heartbeat present. Arrows, 1: embryo, 2: yolk sac, 3: embryonic vesicle, 4: fundouterine, 5: empty endometrial cavity.

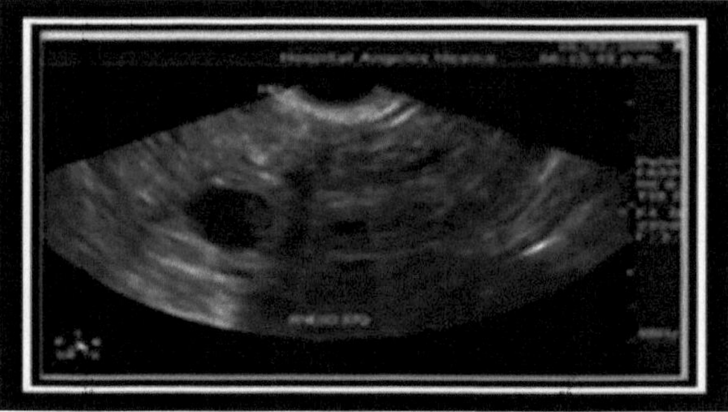

Cystic image in annexe with echoes within it

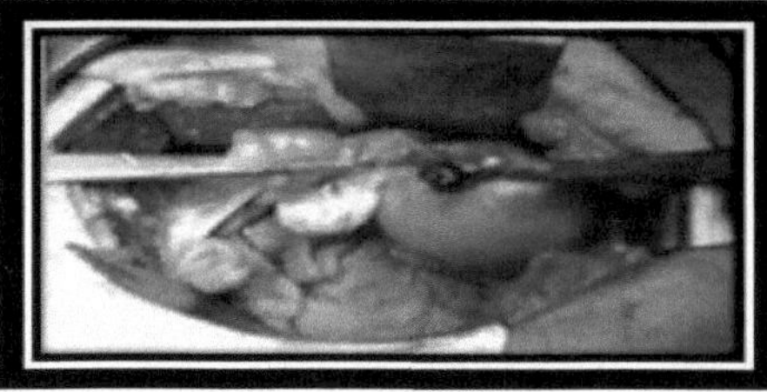

Left Ectopic Anatomical Pregnancy Anatomical Part

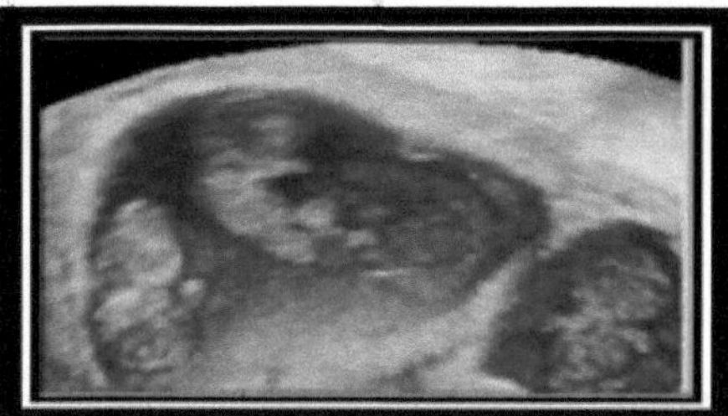

Twin Pregnancy

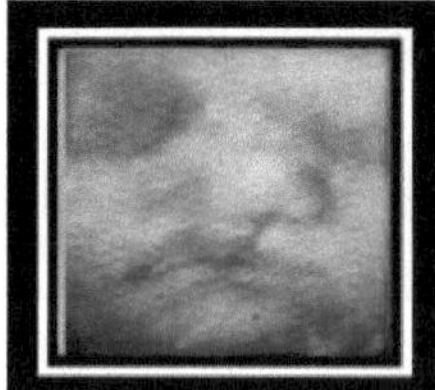 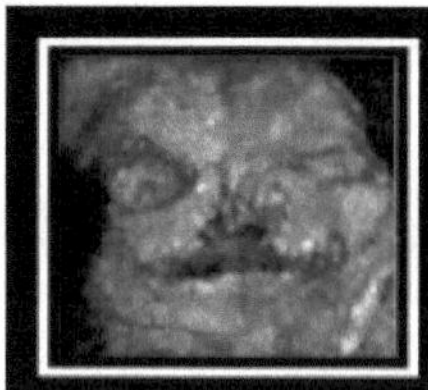

Cleft lip

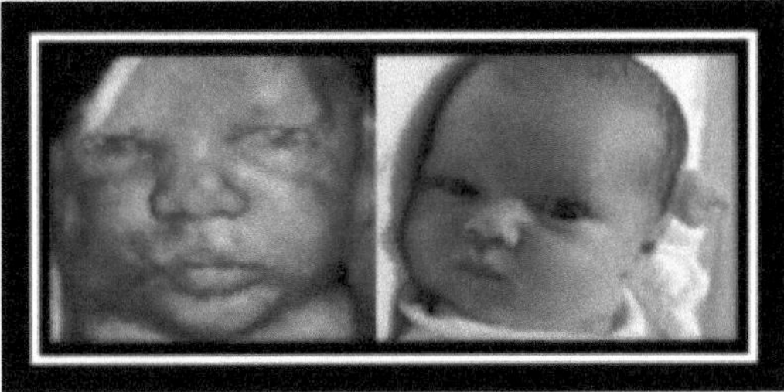

Macizo Facial normal

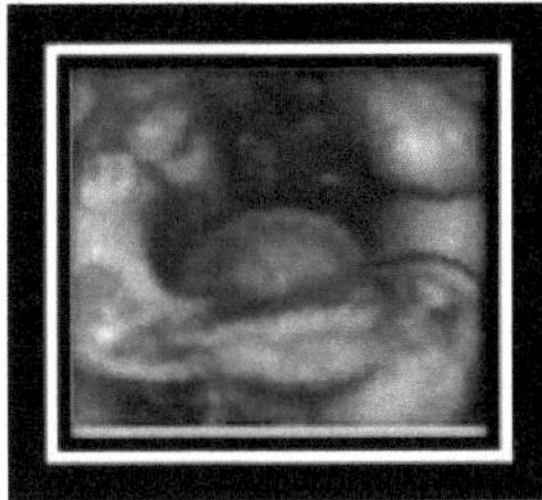
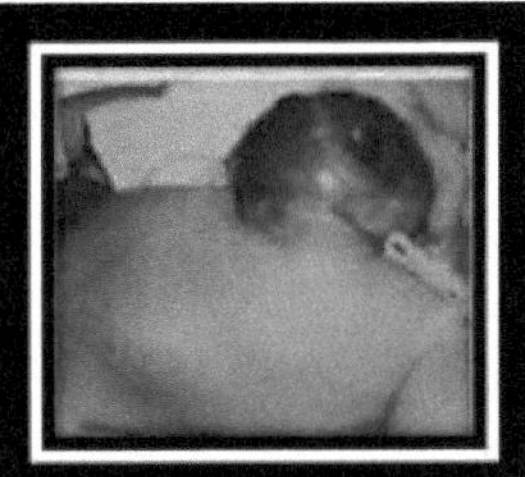

Onfalocele

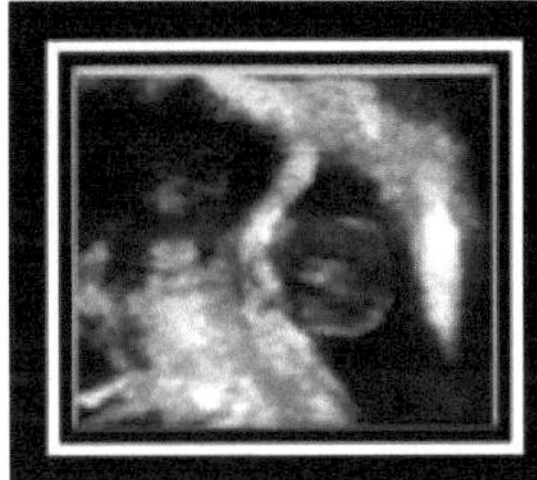
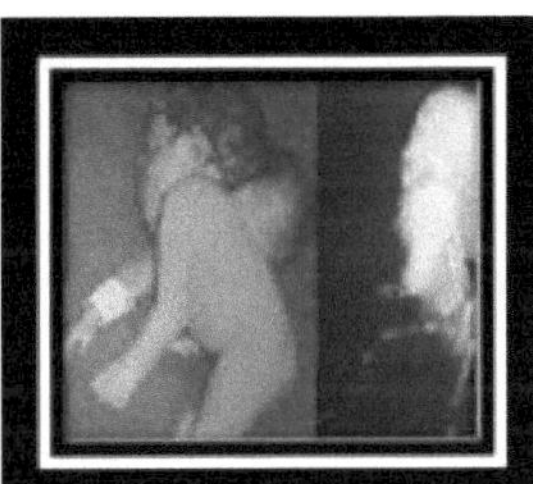

Mielomeningocele
**Normal Facial Mass
Omphalocele
Myelomeningocele**

Chapter 13

Obstetric ultrasound and fetal biometry.

Introduction.

There are two moments when its high value has been noted.
- Between 18 and 22 weeks from the first day of the last menstrual period.
- Between 32 and 36 weeks from the first day of the last menstrual period.

Indications for obstetric US.

(Before 18 - 22 Weeks).

There is no real indication of US in the first trimester unless there is a clinical reason; however, there is no real indication of US in the second trimester unless there is a clinical reason:
- 90% of foetal malformations occur without a family history.
- Fetal malformations may be present in the presence of a clinically normal pregnancy.
- Neither the clinical examination nor the family history can suggest multiple pregnancy.
- Many women with placenta praevia have no clinical manifestations until labour begins.
- Most women do not know the exact date of their last menstrual period; a two-week discrepancy is important in case of premature birth.

Importance of obstetric US.

(18 - 22 Weeks).

1   It allows the EG to be established with a fair degree of accuracy.
2   Allows the diagnosis of foetal malformations and multiple pregnancies.
3   Allows the placenta to be located.
4   It allows to recognise myomas or other pelvic masses that may hinder pregnancy.

Importance of obstetric US.

(32 - 36 Weeks).

1   Recognise a CIUR.
2   To recognise foetal malformations not detected in the first US.
3   Confirm fetal presentation and position.
4   Locate the placenta accurately.
5   Determine the amount of LA.
6   To exclude possible complications, fibroids, ovarian tumours, etc.

Preparation and Technique.

In the first few weeks it is essential to carry out the study with a full bladder.

The patient lying supine.

Transverse and longitudinal slices will be made and combined with oblique slices focusing the transducer from right to left and vice versa.

Transducers of 3,5 or 5 MHz are used.

Early pregnancy.

It is based on the location of the OS, which can be identified at 6 weeks of amenorrhoea, with visualisation of a double echogenic ring in the uterus. The inner ring of uniform echogenicity, 2 mm thick or slightly thicker, and on the outside, another echogenic ring which does not completely surround the OS and represents the uterus. These echogenic rings are separated by an anechogenic space representing the residual endometrial cavity.

At 5 to 6 weeks the largest diameter of the OS is between 1 and 2 cm. At 8 weeks the OS occupies half of the uterus; at 9 weeks it occupies two thirds of the uterus and at 10 weeks it fills the uterus completely.

The EG can be calculated from the size of the SG. For this purpose, a sagittal and a 90-degree cross-section are taken. The average SG measurement is the sum of these measurements divided by 3.

$$\frac{\text{Length} + \text{AP} + \text{Width}}{3} = \text{corresponding boards.}$$

IUD.

The US allows its identification and localisation within or outside the uterus, which can reach the splenic area or the vagina. The possibility of a well-placed IUD and simultaneous pregnancy should make us consider a future abortion.

Ectopic pregnancy.

Ectopic pregnancy is considered to be the implantation of the fertilised lobule or blastocyst outside the endometrial cavity, frequently its location is tubal and in the ampullary or ^stmic portion of the tubes for 98%, 60% are ampullary, 30% ^stmic, 5% ffmbrical, 3% intertitial and only the remaining 2% correspond to other ovarian locations which can be ovarian, cervical, intraligamentary and primitive abdominal. Ectopic pregnancy is known as the great simulator of obstetrics and gynaecology because of its various clinical manifestations, with different symptoms and signs. Depending on the course of the pregnancy, it can be divided into two groups.

> Uncomplicated Ectopic Pregnancy
> Complicated Ectopic Pregnancy

Signs and symptoms:

> Menstrual delay and irregularity
> Subjective symptoms of pregnancy
> Pain
> Adnexal tumour
> Uterus with signs of pregnancy

Risk Groups

> History of pelvic inflammation, especially Chlamydia Trach and Trichomona Neuseria gonorrheae (gonorrhoea).
> Tubal operations to search for fertility
> Previous ectopic pregnancy
> Tubaric Sterilisation
> Patients with intrauterine devices
> Ingestion of oral devices.
> Pregnancy by assisted reproduction techniques
> Smoking

The patient should come with a full bladder, which is necessary for:

> To create a sonic window that allows a good delimitation of the pelvic structures.
> Elevate or displace neighbouring pelvic bowel loops.
> To assess the echogenicity of a pelvic mass under study with bladder sonolucency.

When interpreting a gynaecological ultrasound or suspected first trimester ectopic pregnancy, it is necessary to first identify the main anatomical structures, especially the uterus and adnexal structures.

Under normal conditions and in a CL, the uterus appears to be located behind the bladder with the fundus slightly anterior to the neck except in cases of retroversion. In tubal ectopic pregnancy, the fertilised ovum implants below the epithelium, forming a fluid-filled SG surrounded by trophoblastic tissue that extends along the thin wall of the tube, favouring its distension and rupture.

	Not broken	Broken
Suggestive signs	1- Absence of intrauterine SG.	1. ^dem 1. Mixed or echodense masses,

Diagnostic signs	2- Complex adnexal mass, expression of SG or products of conception 3- Presence of foetal mobility 4- No intraperitoneal free Kquido 5- Enlarged uterus with decidual reaction	in the Douglas pouch, representing ruptured SG or haematomas. 2. No foetal mobility 4- Presence of peritoneal free Kquides 5- Uterine enlargement with decidual reaction 6- Displacement of uterus by a complex adnexal mass.

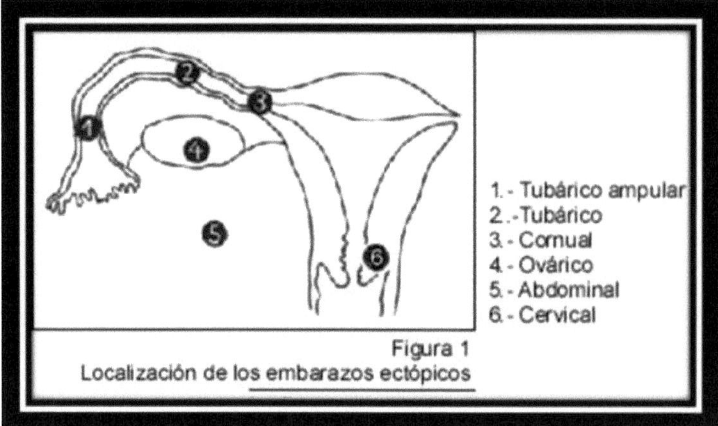

Figura 1
Localización de los embarazos ectópicos

Embryo.
Although the OS can be recognised between 5 and 6 weeks, the embryo is not visible until 7 weeks, in the form of an echogenic area, located eccentrically in the OS, in which the LCs are identified.
Between 9 and 10 weeks the head is identified and movements are seen.
From 11 weeks onwards the skull is visible.

Saco Vitelino.
From 7 weeks onwards, the SV is visualised as a rounded cystic image, 4 to 5 mm in size, next to the foetus and where the formation of blood cells begins.
At 11 weeks it should disappear. Not to be confused with a GS, it is not always present.

Multiple pregnancy.
The earliest time to recognise it is at 8 weeks, but the patient should never be informed unless both embryos or foetuses are seen, which is assured between 14 and 18 weeks.

First Trimester Disturbances.
1   Small SG. It is almost always an expression of anembryonic gestation. Not seen the foetus and the SG is smaller. If in doubt, repeat the examination.
2   Fetal death or miscarriage. There is almost always a history of bleeding or colic. The uterus may appear normal, small or enlarged (if there is intrauterine haematoma). The fetal pole can be seen but there is no cardiac activity. Repeat the

examination if in doubt.

3   Saco vacte. There is a history of amenorrhoea and metrorrhagia. When the picture is recent, the uterus appears enlarged, but vacuolated.

4   Incomplete abortion. The clinical picture is quite suggestive, the uterus appears empty and the endometrial canal may appear normal. If the abortion is incomplete, the uterus appears smaller with a very deformed OS and an amorphous content, of very variable size, shape and echogenicity, an expression of the retention of blood and placenta. The possibility of a mole must always be excluded.

Uterus enlarged.

An enlarged uterus at the time of pregnancy should be ruled out:

1   Hydatidiform mole. The uterus appears enlarged, filled with a mass of uniform echoes resembling a "snowstorm", with cystic spaces. It may or may not be associated with pregnancy and in these cases there is an increased incidence of chromosomal disorders.

2   Choriocarcinoma. It should be suspected when a mole is thought to be present and the uterus is very enlarged and there are large areas of necrosis and haemorrhage inside the uterus.

3   Intrauterine haemorrhage due to abortion. It is accompanied by bleeding. US shows intrauterine blood separating the chorio-amniotic membrane from the decidua, which shows a well-defined anechogenic area. The blood may be anechogenic, hyperechogenic or mixed. Fetal vitality should be identified.

4   Large or irregular uterus. In the first trimester it is very suggestive of a fibroid and must be measured and located. It must be differentiated from uterine contraction and areas of necrosis are frequent.

Obstetric study algorithm.

Obstetric examination.

Fetal biometry.

Length Corona-Rabadilla.

It is the most accurate parameter for the determination of foetal age up to 11 weeks. Subsequently, given the curvature of the foetus, this measurement is affected and from 12 weeks onwards the DBP is more accurate.

The maximum longitudinal diameter of the embryo is measured from the cephalic pole to the outer surface of the buttocks. The amniotic sac and the foetal limbs must not be included.

Fetal biometry.

Measurement of DBP.

It is the ideal method for fetal age determination between 12 and 26 weeks. The DBP is the distance between the parietal eminences on both sides of the skull. For this purpose a cross section of the skull must be obtained, which is recognised by the ovoid shape of the skull and by the interruption of the mid-echo of the brain sickle produced by the cavum of the septum pellucidum and the thalamus. Measurement is made from the outer table of the proximal portion of the skull to the inner table of the distal portion of the skull. The PB should not be included.

Fetal biometry.

Fronto-Occipital Diameter Measurement.

It is measured along the major axis of the skull at the level of the sickle lhea, from the frontal prominence to the occipital prominence.

DBP, DFO and CH must be measured together to obtain an average calculation.

Fetal biometry.

Mdice Cefalico.

BPD is a fairly reliable method for the determination of gestational age, except when the head is deformed or there is an alteration of the intracranial contents. In these cases the IC is of great value.

CI = $\underline{DBP}$ x 100 normal: 70-86 (± 2DS).
DFO

Fetal biometry.
Head circumference index.

If the BF is within the normal range, DBP is of great value in determining the EG. If the BF is outside the normal range (less than 70 or greater than 86), BPD measurement should not be used to calculate GA. Instead, head circumference measurement should be used.

CC = DBP + DOF x 1.57 = 70-86

Fetal biometry.
Abdominal circumference.

It is used for the study of intrauterine growth disorders. The measurement is made at the level of the foetal umbilical portion of the left PV at the moment it enters the liver. In a cut at this level, the AP and transverse diameters should be measured.

CA = DAP + DT x 1.75

Normal (see tables)

Decreased CA | 5th percentile

Increased CA $ 95 percentile

Fetal biometry.
Measurement of long bones.

HLs can be identified from 13 weeks onwards. A longitudinal section of the LH to be studied should be obtained and measured from the distal to the proximal portions. Measurement of the LH and mainly the femur allows a fairly accurate determination of the EG, especially in cases of intracranial pathology.

The DLF should be compared with the DBP or with the EG.

It can be said to be normal when the figure falls within the 2DS for a given EG. It is proportional to the DBP if the DLF measurement falls within 2DS of the DBP. A femur is said to be even smaller or 5 mm smaller than 2DS below the mean.

Caution: There are limits to the accuracy of US in fetal biometry.

- Clinical and laboratory findings should be included.

-Measurements should be made when in doubt.

Serially at intervals of 2 to 3 weeks, the check-up should not be weekly as the changes are usually discrete.

Recognition of CIUR.

A distinction must be made between a symmetric and an asymmetric CIUR.

1 Symmetrical or low profile foetus. The growth retardation is caused by chromosomal abnormalities, infections or poor maternal nutrition and manifests early in gestation. The head-to-body ratio remains within the normal range and the foetus is symmetrically retarded, i.e. all measurements appear reduced in the same proportion.

2 Asymmetrical ICUR. The abdominal circumference is below normal and the head-body ratio is abnormal. This is due to placental insufficiency in the mother with pre-eclampsia. The prognosis can be improved with appropriate treatment.

Gestational Age Determination.

Comparison of fetal size and GA can never be a valuable indicator in CIUR.

Therefore, GD should be defined early by determining crown-rump diameter, fetal head measurement and femoral length, all in the first US study.

Measurement of DBP or CF is appropriate for the calculation of estimated GA.

If DBP alone is used, 60% of growth disorders are detected. But when combined with other measurements the sensitivity rises to 70-80%.

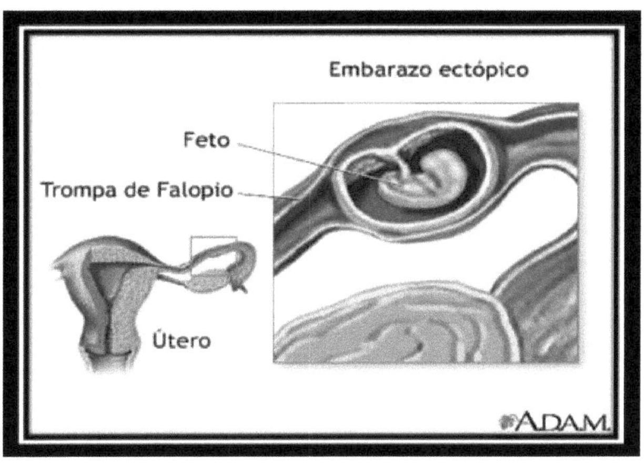

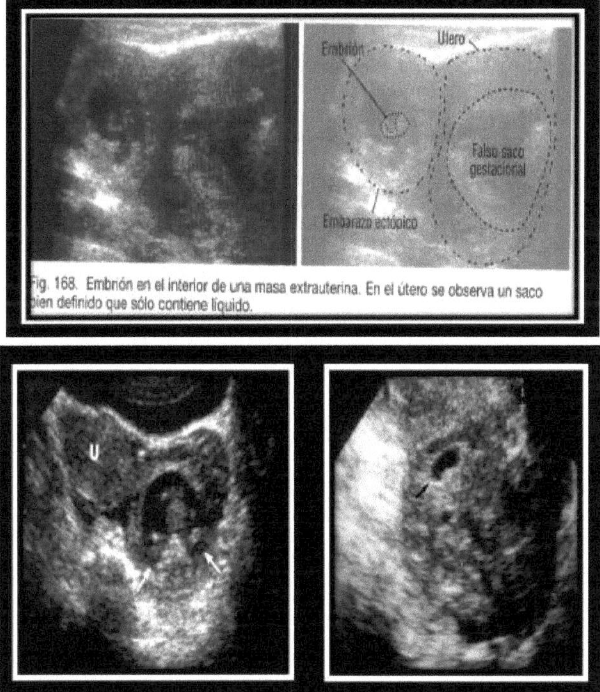

Fig. 168. Embrión en el interior de una masa extrauterina. En el útero se observa un saco bien definido que sólo contiene líquido.

Ectopic pregnancy is the failure of a fertilised egg to reach the endometrial cavity of the uterus.

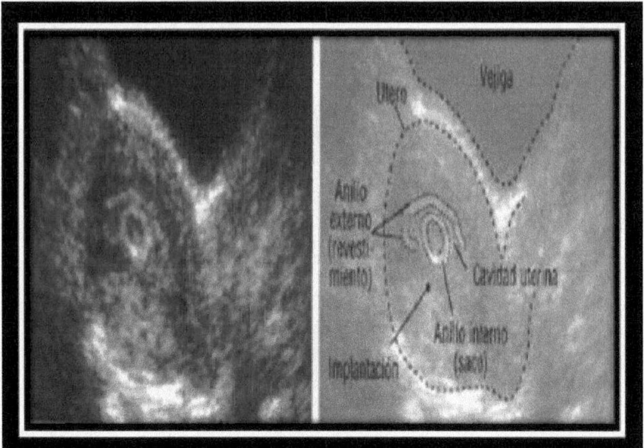

5 to 6 weeks gestational sac

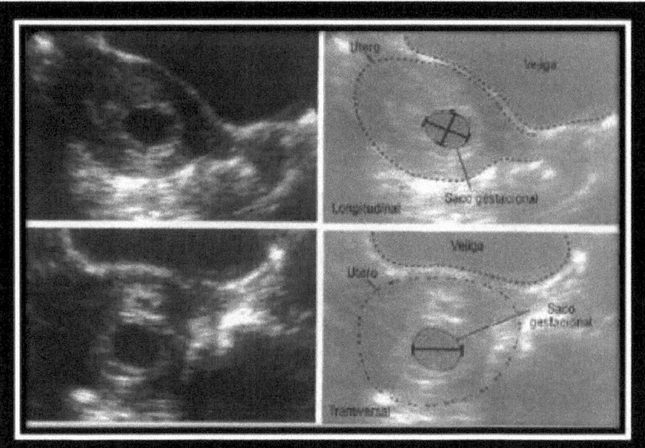

Medición del saco gestacional

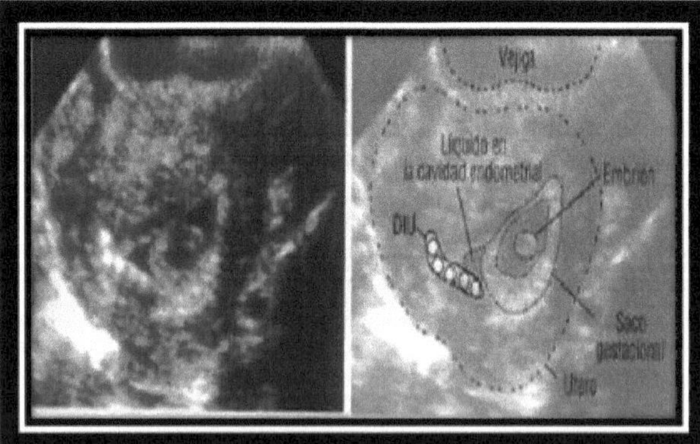

Embarazo con DIU

Measurement of the gestational sac

Pregnancy with an IUD

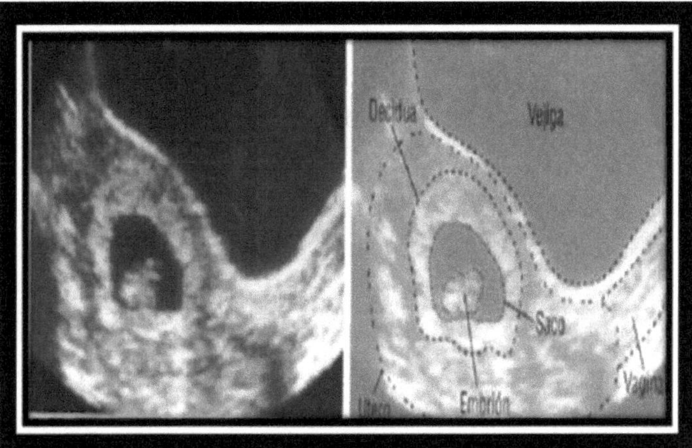

9 Weeks

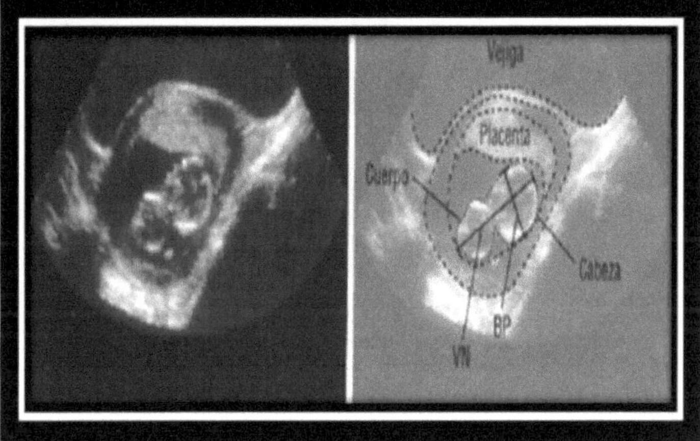

12 Weeks

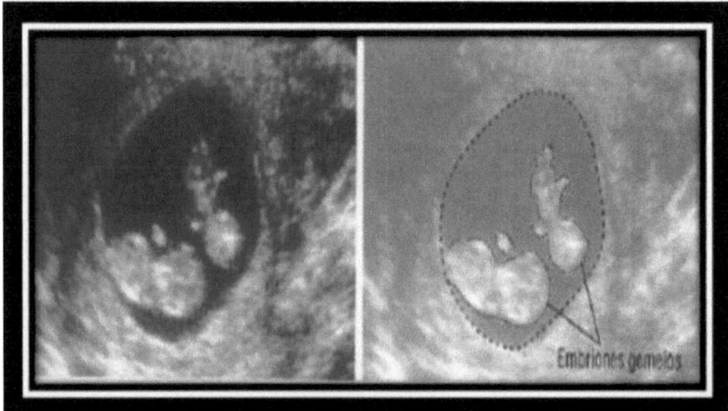

Twin pregnancy

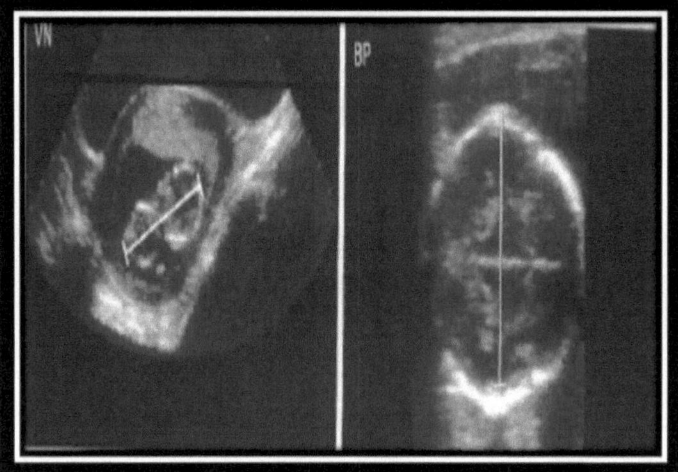

11 Weeks pregnant

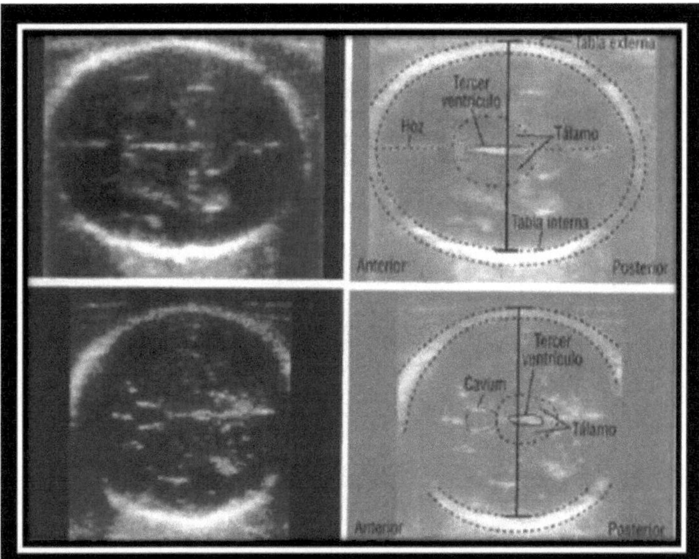

Fetal skull at 24 weeks

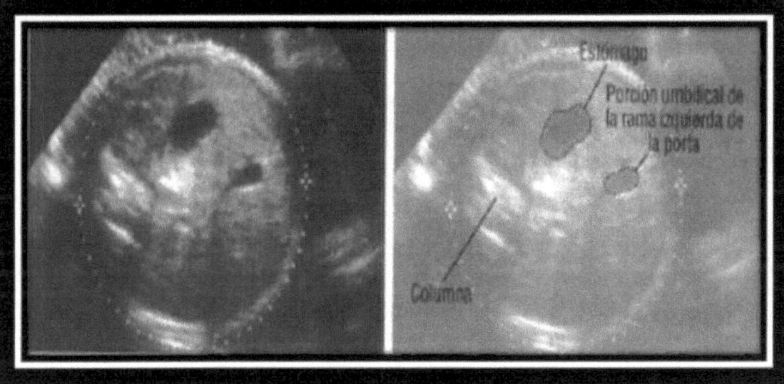

Abdominal perimeter

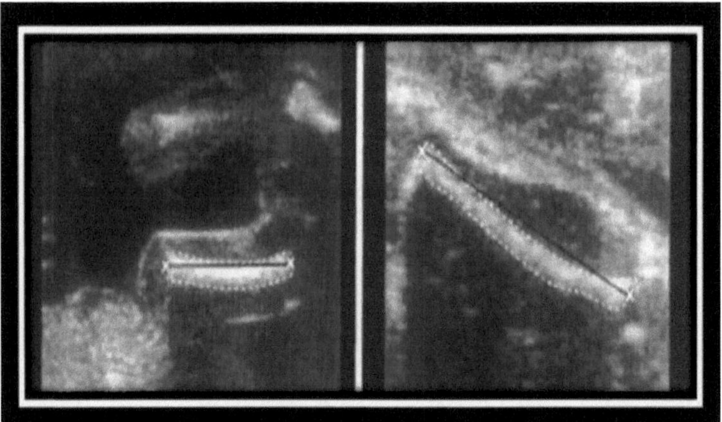

Femur length

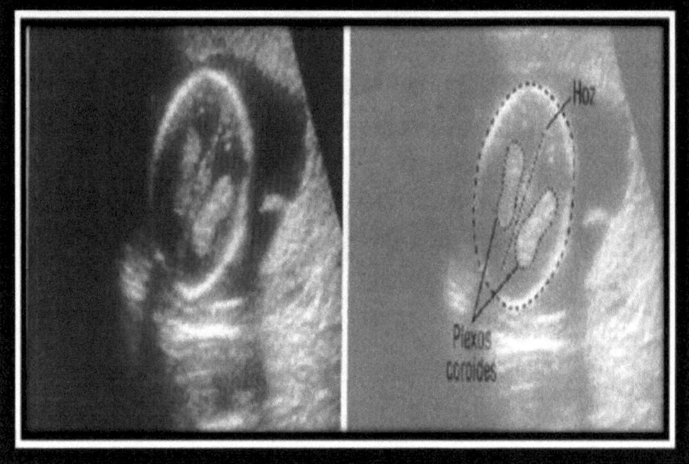

Axial imaging 17 weeks

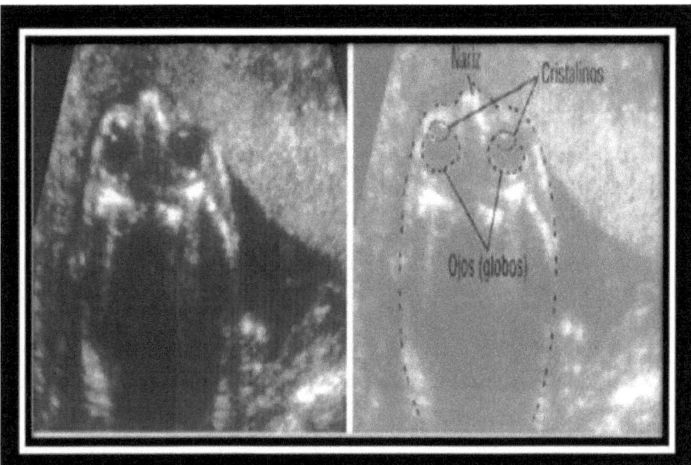

Axial image of the orbits

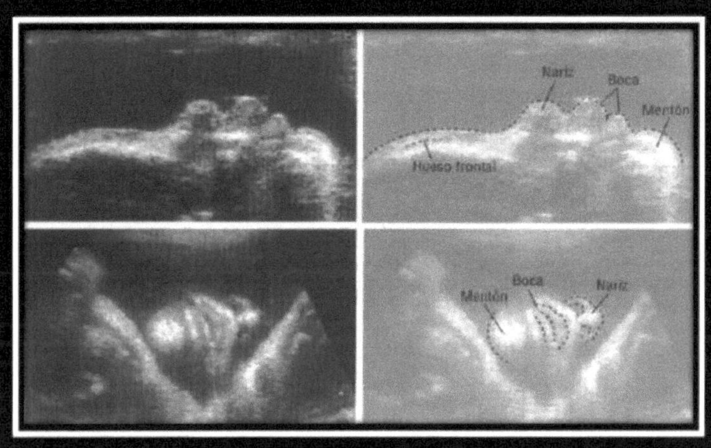

Sagittal and coronal image

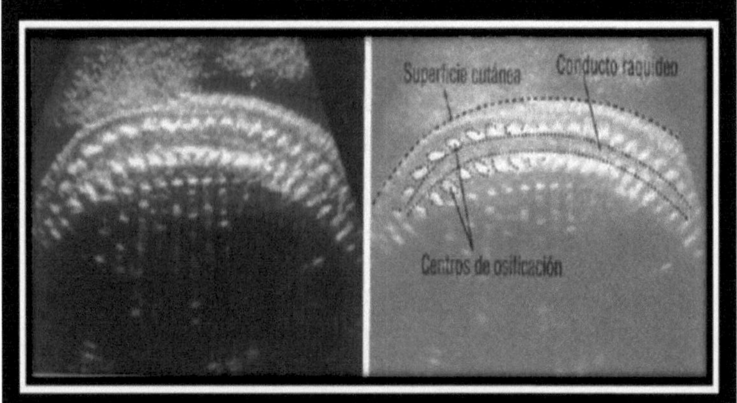

Longitudinal image 22 weeks Column

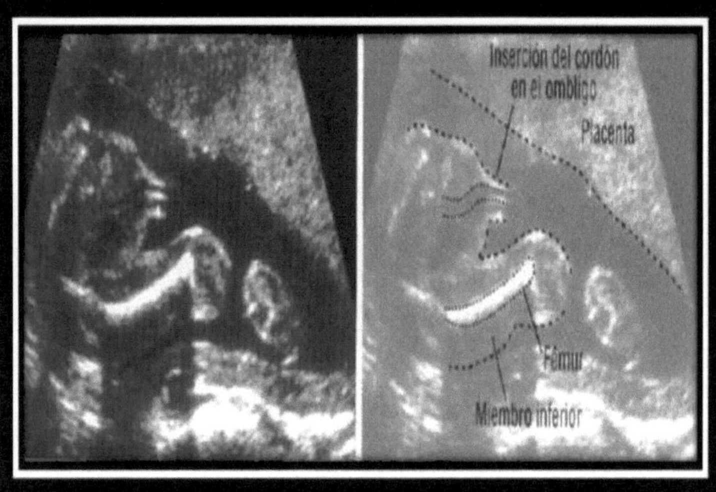

Umbilical Cord

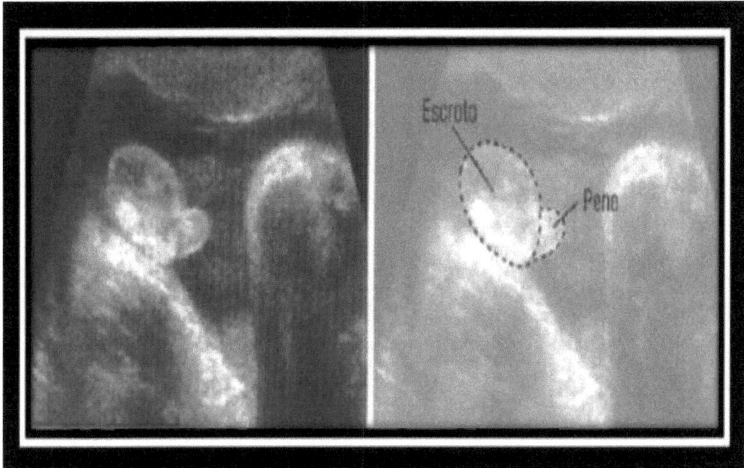

Male genitalia 23 weeks

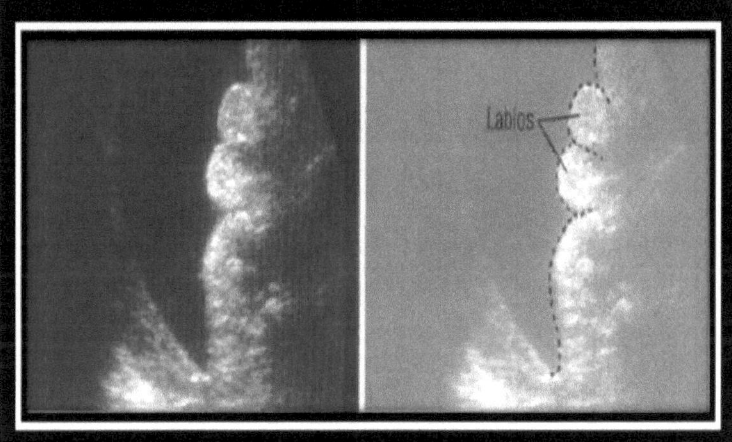

Female genitalia 28 weeks

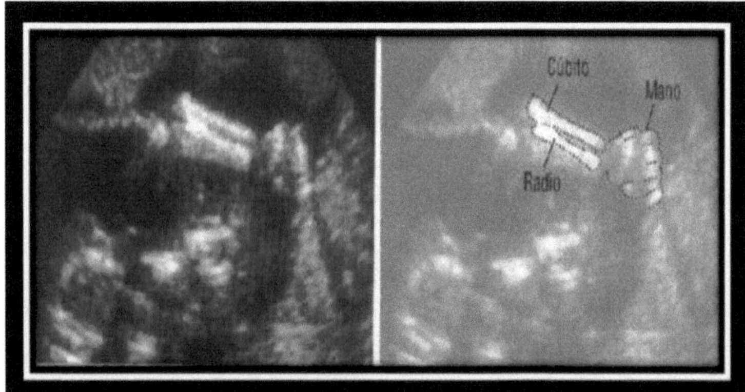

Arms and hands

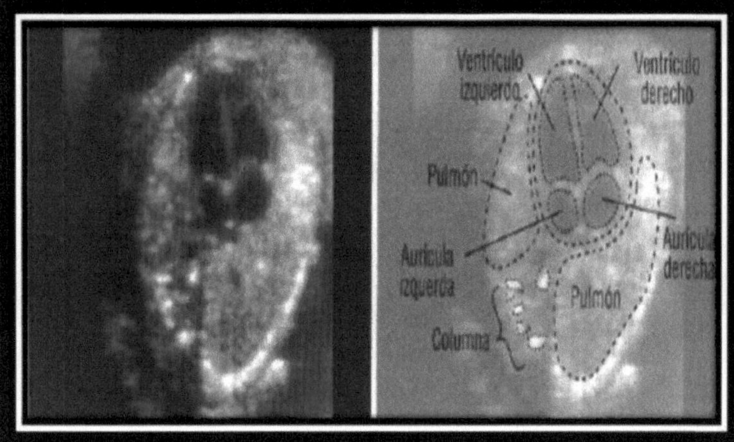

Heart and lung of a foetus

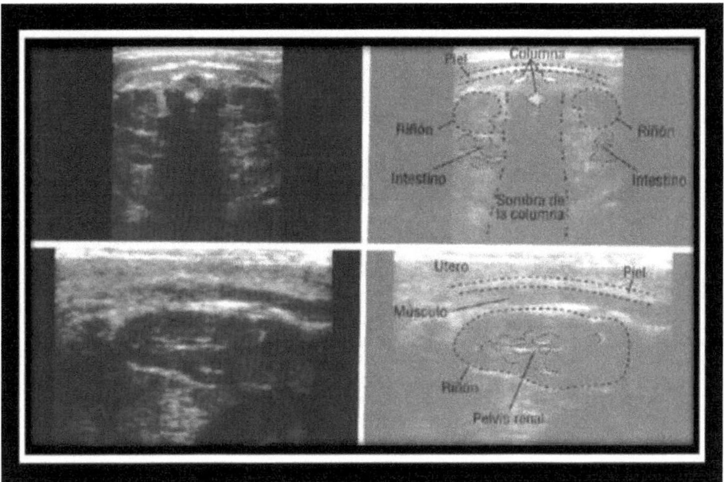

Rinon
"1st Quarter Anomalies

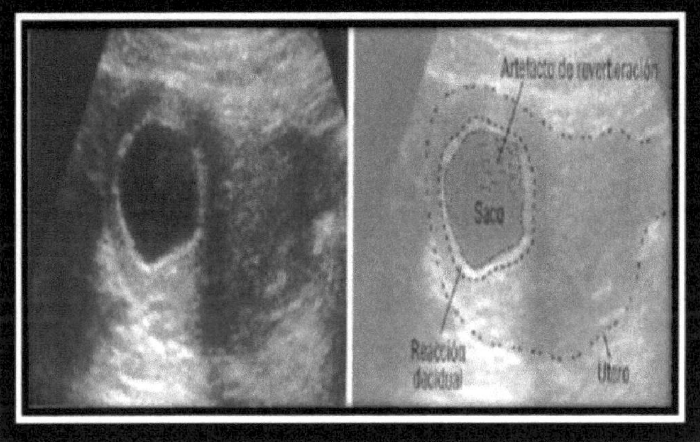

Non-embryonic egg

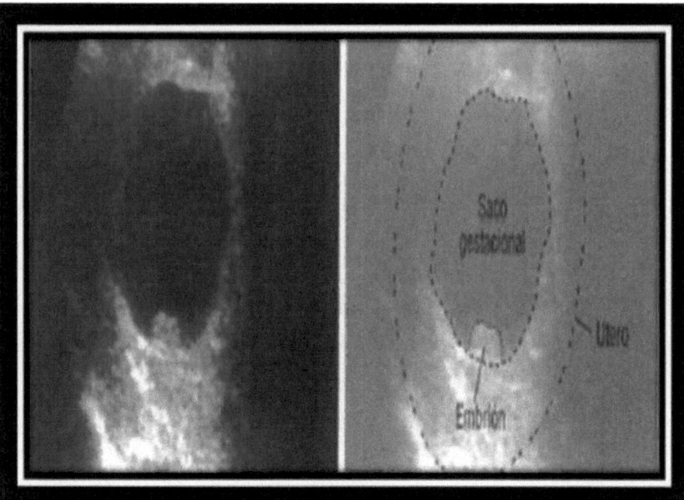

Stillbirth

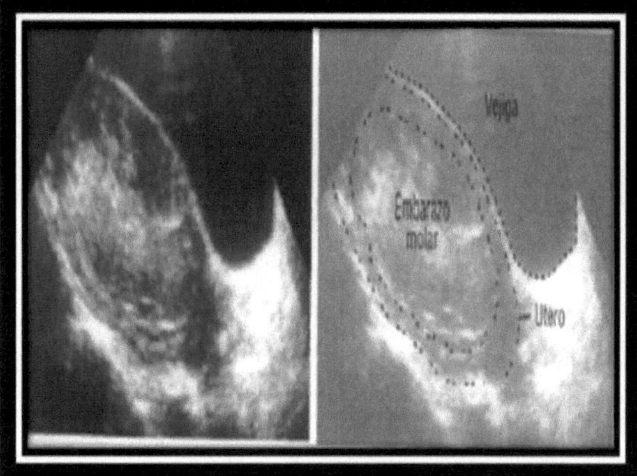

Molar Pregnancy

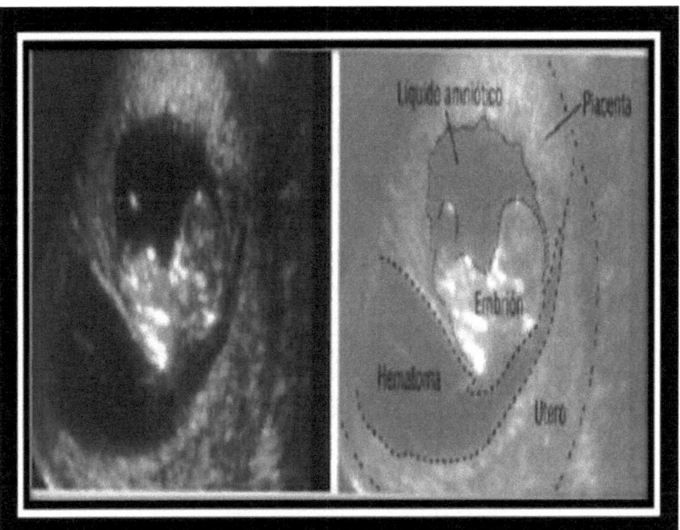

Intrauterine haematoma

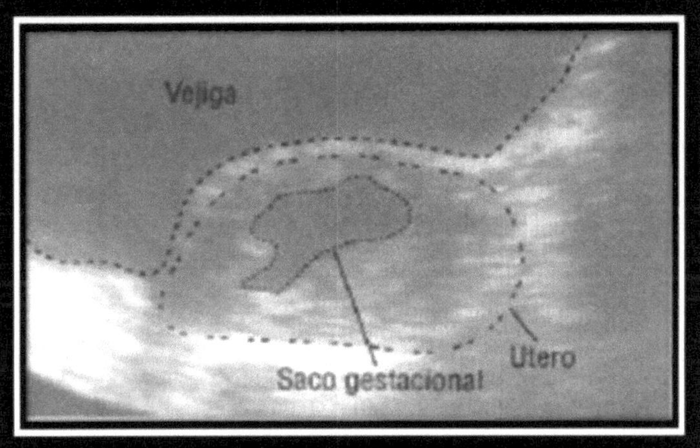

Incomplete abortion

Chapter 14

Scrotal and Testicular Ultrasound.

Indications for US of the scrotum and testicles.

1   Inflammation of the scrotum.
2   Scrotal trauma.
3   Testicular infections.
4   Acute or sub-acute pain.
5   Testicular absence.
6   Haematospermia.
7   Infertility.

Preparation and Technique.

The testicular US study does not require prior preparation, and the study is performed with high frequency linear transducers (7.5 MHz, 10 MHz).

The penis is placed over the pubis (upwards) and covered by a drape, the patient is asked to lift the scrotal pouch and close the legs or they may be slightly spread apart. Cross-sections are made from top to bottom and longitudinal sections from outside to inside. The study is always comparative.

Testicular anatomy.

The testis is oval, homogeneous and hyperechogenic.

Its average adult length is 5 cm, its width is 3 cm and its transverse diameter is 2 cm^ as well as its vertical diameter is 2.5 cm.

The epididymis is located on the posterior aspect of the testis and is more echogenic. It is divided into head, body and tail. The two testis are separated at the medial side of the scrotum by a hyperechogenic septum. Sometimes there may be a small collection of kquid.

In the normal testis, the fibrous mediastinum (more echogenic) and the tunica albughea can be identified.

Testicular venous drainage is carried out through a superficial and a deep venous system, almost all of which is produced by the latter.

Deep venous system: Anterior venous group of the pampiniform plexus, consisting of the deep spermatic (inter lobular) veins which join the tributary veins of the epididymal head to form the anterior group of the pampiniform plexus which ascends the anterior aspect of the spermatic cord, giving rise to the internal spermatic vein; The right vein empties into the anterior aspect of the vena cava about two centimetres from the junction with the renal vein, and the left into the homolateral renal vein.

Superficial venous system: Posterior group of the pampiniform plexus, the veins of the body and the tail of the epididymis with the network of the vas deferens itself, form the posterior group of the pampiniform plexus in which the external spermatic vein and the vein of the vas deferens can be distinguished. The external spermatic vein, which receives the veins of the cremasteric plexus, flows into the epigastric, the branch of the external iliac and the vena deferentia flows into the hypogastric.

The veins of the anterior and posterior group of the pampiniform plexus are anastomosed to each other by numerous communications, which may sometimes explain the persistence of varicocele after treatment.

Pathological alterations.

(Hernia).

It is a hernia of the omentum, mesentery or bowel loops often associated with hydrocele. The loops appear as complex masses or as hypoechogenic areas. If a hernia is suspected, a valsalva manoeuvre should be performed.

Pathological alterations.

(Torsion of the testicular appendix).

Torsion of testicular appendages is an obligatory differential diagnosis in acute pain with or without inflammation; it is usually unilateral although synchronous torsion has been described, is most common between 7 and 12 years but can occur in adults.

Four possible intrascrotal appendages can become twisted: The testicular appendix or hydatid of Morgagni, a remnant of the Mullerian ducts and accounts for 92% of torsions; the appendix of the head of the epid^dymus, a Wolffian remnant and contributes 7% of torsions; the organ of Giraldes, also called parad^dymus or "innominate organ", a Wolffian remnant, at 0.7% and the vas aberrans which is a mesonephric remnant located at the junction between the body and tail of the epididymis at 0.3%.

Pathological alterations.
(Epididymitis).
The epididymis appears thickened and hypoechogenic. Sometimes it is associated with orchitis and the testis becomes hypo- or hyperechogenic, the latter pattern often reflecting the degree of chronicity of the inflammatory process.

Pathological alterations.
(Orchitis).
Orchitis is characterised by being accompanied by a clinical picture of significant pain, this being the most significant symptom. On ultrasonographic study we will find localised or diffuse areas where there is a decrease in testicular echogenicity. Occasionally, orchitis evolves leaving fibrous processes in its wake, which will be observed as echogenic images in the testicular parenchyma.

Pathological alterations.
(Cyst of the epididymis or testis).
Epididymal cysts can be single or multiple, they must be differentiated from the varicoceles.

Although testicular cysts are infrequent, they can also be found with clear, thin-walled contents.

Pathological alterations.
(Hydrocele).
It may be anechogenic and clear in content or it may present internal echoes showing cellularity due to inflammation or trauma, in some cases it is not uncommon to find the presence of septa.

Hydroceles can frequently occur as post-surgical complications of varicocele.

Pathological alterations.
(Varicocele).
Multiple, tortuous, tubular hypoechogenic structures are seen around the periphery of the testis. They are more frequent on the left side and are associated with infertility in a considerable number of patients. It must be differentiated from a spermatocele which is not modified by valsalva manoeuvres.

Varicoceles can occur extratesticularly (the most frequent) or intratesticularly (less frequent).

Pathological alterations.
(Spermatocele).
It is an intraparenchymal cystic lesion of the testis, adjacent to the testicular mediastinum, in the area of the testicular network, which communicates with the seminiferous tubules, which differentiates it from ectasia of the rete testis, in which there is no communication with the seminiferous tubules, containing spermatozoa in its interior.

Pathological alterations.
(Testicular trauma).
After trauma, the testicle may be normal in size and appearance or enlarged,

sometimes with the presence of hydrocele, and may show complex echogenicity due to haematoma. Sometimes it is found surrounding the testis, a haematocele, or it may present as an intratesticular haematoma, with partial or total rupture of the testis.

Pathological testicular disorders.
(Atrophy).
It is usually a testicular condition secondary to direct trauma to the testicle, varicocele, orchitis or following testicular torsion and whose diagnosis and treatment was not made in a timely manner. Testicular atrophy occurs in one third of adolescents who develop orchitis caused by mumps. On ultrasound, the testicles appear asymmetrical, reduced in size, with alteration of the testicles.
in the echogenicity of the parenchyma (hypoechogenic).

Pathological testicular disorders.
(Calcifications).
Calcifications can be extratesticular (scrolites) or intratesticular (parenchymal calcifications), they are benign lesions, but an important group of authors consider that in a patient with parenchymal microcalcifications it is advisable to carry out evolutionary ultrasonographic studies as they can be an indicative sign of possible future malignant lesions.

Pathological testicular disorders.
(Abscesses).
Abscesses begin as common inflammatory processes that for multiple reasons follow a torpid evolution as a result of the infectious process that is established in it. They can develop as a consequence of surgical interventions, trauma with intratesticular bleeding or injuries that produce rupture of the scrotal skin, among other causes.
In ecograffa they will be visualised as complex mixed processes.

Pathological alterations.
(Tumours).
As in the rest of the body, testicular tumours are classified as follows:
- Benign and
- Evil.

ANATOMOPATHOLOGICAL CLASSIFICATION OF TESTICULAR TUMOURS (WHO).
1.- Germ cell tumours:
A.- Tumours with a single histological pattern (60%)
Seminoma: Upic, classic, anaplastic, spermatocystic.
Embryonal carcinoma.
Yolk sac tumour (embryonal carcinoma of infantile type or endodermal sinus tumour).
Polyembryoma.
Choriocarcinoma.
Mature teratoma or with malignant transformation.
B.- Tumours with more than one histological pattern (40%)
Embryonal carcinoma with teratoma (teratocarcinoma).
Choriocarcinoma associated with any of the other types.
Other combinations (specify type).
2.- Tumours of the sexual cords and gonadal stroma.
A.- Well-differentiated forms:
Leydig cell tumours.
Sertoli cell tumours.
Granulosa cell tumours.
B.- Mixed forms.

Incompletely differentiated forms.
3. Non-specialised testicular stromal tumours.
Angiomas.
Leiomyomas.
Neurofibromas.
Sarcomas.
Carcinoids.
4. Metastatic or secondary tumours.
Lymphoma.
Leukaemia.
Metastasis.
Plasmacytoma.
Pathological alterations.
(Pseudotumours).
They are also known as fibrous periorchitis, non-spermatocytic paratesticular fibrosis, granulomatous periorchitis or reactive periorchitis. They are mobile masses within the tunica vaginalis with the presence of one or more nodules. When large, they simulate a tumour even if there is a history of infection or previous trauma. The masses are composed of hyalinised collagen and granulation tissue with extensive calcifications.
Pathological alterations.
(Malignant tumours).
Intratesticular neoplasms constitute 1% to 2% of all malignant pathologies in men, are more frequent in whites and are the fifth most frequent cause of death in males between 15 and 34 years of age.
They occur at a frequency of 2 per 100,000 men and the incidence is highest in the 15-34 age group.
The cause of testicular neoplasms is still unknown, but congenital factors (family history in up to 16%, cryptorchid testis, etc.) and acquired factors (trauma and infection) have been proposed.
Between 65% to 94% present as a painless testicular mass or diffuse testicular enlargement and about 4% to 14% present with symptoms of metastatic disease.
Pathological testicular disorders.
(Metastasis).
In a small percentage of cases, however, the testis and/or epididymis can also be the site of metastases from neighbouring organs, or from lymphomatous infiltration in the course of leukaemias.

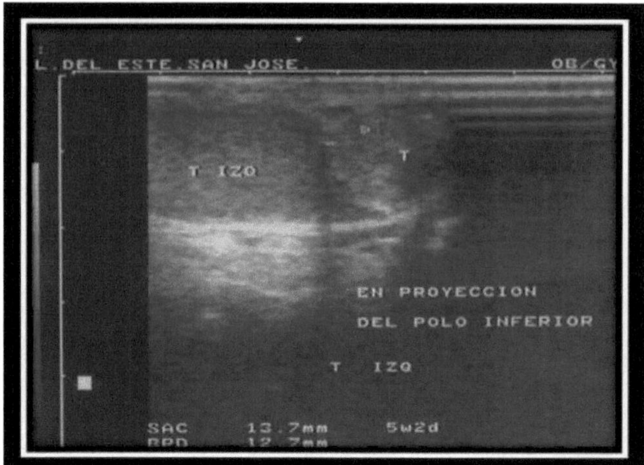

T projecting towards the inferior pole of the left testicle at the level of the tail of the epididymis.

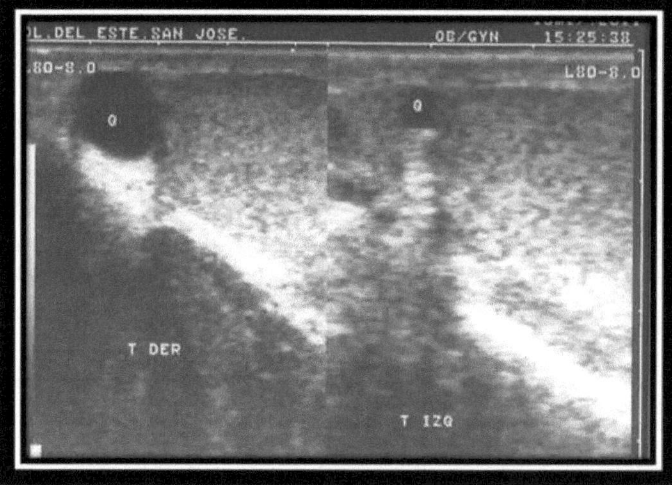

Left testicular atrophy and liquid collection bordering it in relation to hydrocele.

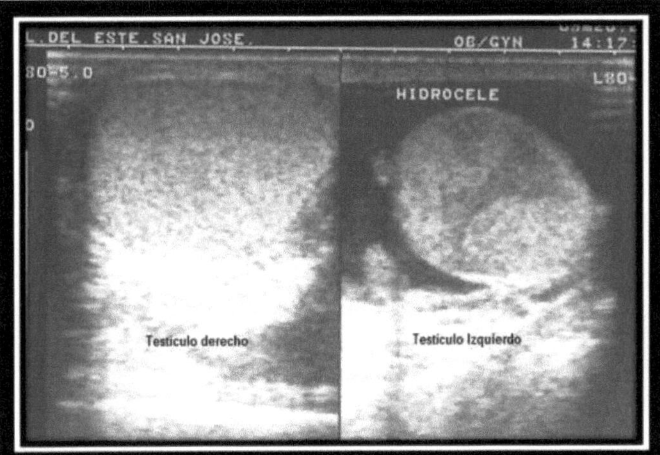

Anechoic image of well-defined contours projecting towards the head of the right and left epididymis with cyst-like appearance.

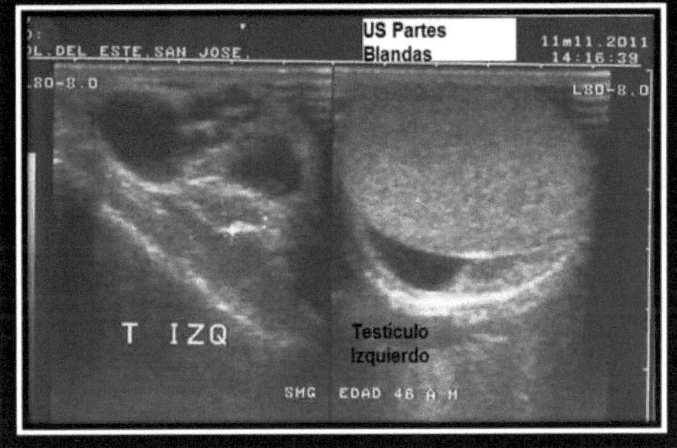

Complex projection image of the left epididymal head, composite ultrasonographic image.

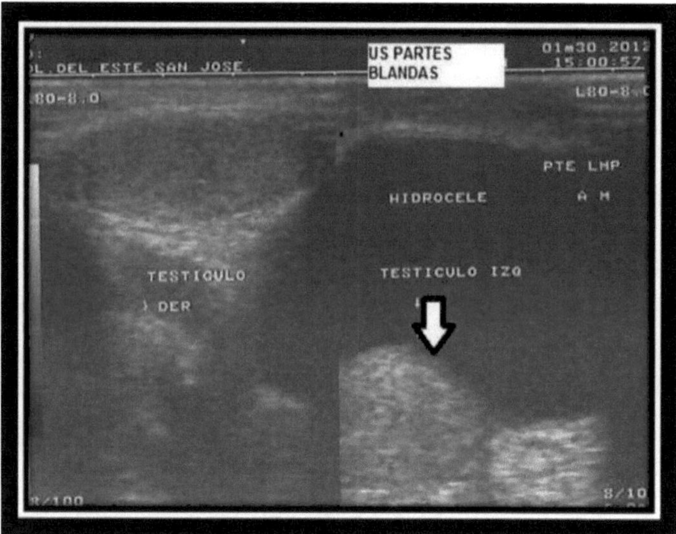

Marked liquid collection bordering left testicle, hydrocele.

Chapter 15

Ultrasound of thyroid and neck vessels.
Thyroid gland.

Indications for Thyroid US.

1 Palpable nodule or enlargement in the anterior neck region.
2 Progressive control of adenomas and hyperplasia.
3 Assessment of surgical remains.
4 Suspected hyperparathyroidism.
5 Search for occult neoplasms or metastases.
6 Pathologies of the upper aerodigestive tract.
7 Staging of tumours in the region.
8 To assess possible sequelae in patients with a history of radiation treatment to the neck.
9 As a guide for BAAF.

Preparation and Technique.

No prior preparation is required.

The study is performed with the patient in the supine decubitus position with a pillow placed behind the shoulders to elevate them and make the head rest on the bed to achieve a hyperextension of the neck.

For the study of the vessels of the neck it is advisable to give a discreet obliquity to the neck.

Transverse, sagittal and oblique slices are performed using 7 MHz or 10 MHz transducers.

Normal anatomy of the neck.

• **Neck vessels**: Includes the CCA and its branches which appear as anechogenic tubular structures with echogenic walls located outside the sternocleidomastoid muscle, the VY is of larger calibre with a more external location and is compressed by the pressure of the transducer.

• **Thyroid**: The lobules of the thyroid and the isthmus have a homogeneous structure, with smooth borders. It is 15 to 20 mm thick, 20 to 25 mm wide and 30 to 50 mm high. In transverse sections it is triangular in shape and in sagittal section each lobule is oval.

• **Muscle**: The most important muscle in the region is the sternocleidomastoid and appears less echogenic than the thyroid.

• **Nodes**: Usually smaller than 1 cm and appear as uniform hypoechogenic structures.

Location and Anatomy of the Thyroid.

• It is located in the anterior region of the neck at the level of the hyoid cartilage.
• Formed by two lobes and an isthmus joining them.
• Both lobules on the sides of the trachea bounded laterally by the arteries carotid, jugular veins and sternocleidomastoid muscles.
• Protected anteriorly by the sternohyoid, sternothyroid and homohyoid muscles.
• Posterior and lateral are the long neck muscles.

Thyroid abnormalities.

• Hemiagenesis.
• Lateral migration of the thyroid.
• Subcutaneous neck mass.
• Thyroglossal duct cyst.

Increase in the volume of the neck.

70% are thyroid nodules and more than 90% are adenomas. Nodules can be malignant and are identifiable on US: hypo- or hyperechogenic, sometimes with cystic components. Benign lesions, however, have fine, sharp, hyperechogenic contours.

Pathological alterations of the thyroid.
(Homogeneous diffuse enlargement).

• They may involve a portion, the whole lobule, the isthmus or both lobes. It is almost always a homogeneous hyperplasia. It may be due to goitre, iodine deficiency, hyperparathyroidism, etc. In acute thyroiditis the thyroid may be hypoechogenic and homogeneous.

Thyroid hyperplasia.

It may be:

J FOCAL

J DIFUSA   (Goitre).

THERE IS FREQUENT PARTICIPATION FROM THE ISTHMUS

Causes of goitre.

• Simple goitre.
• Graves-Basedow disease.
• Acromegaly.
• Lithium treatment.
• Hyperparathyroidism.

US image of goitre.

• Diffuse thyroid enlargement.
• Frequent involvement of the isthmus with diffuse thyroid enlargement.
• Increased thyroid vascularity (Graves-Basedow).
• The thyroid may have an inhomogeneous structure and may develop into a nodular or multinodular goitre.

Thyroiditis.

Caused by: infectious agent or related to autoimmune anomaKas.

• Acute suppurative thyroiditis.
• Postpartum autoimmune thyroiditis.
• Hashimoto's thyroiditis.

By ultrasound:

• Enlargement of the thyroid gland.
• Hypoechogenic thyroid.
• Hypoechogenic foci (suppurative thyroiditis).

Thyroid nodules.

They can be:

• Unique: - Adenoma
- Qusticos
- Carcinoma.
• Multiple: - Adenomatous hyperplasia.

Pathological alterations of the thyroid.
(Heterogeneous enlargement).

• It presents in the form of multiple nodules, solid or complex. In autoimmune thyroiditis it is heterogeneous and resembles a multilocular goitre.

Pathological alterations of the thyroid.
(Localised cystic masses).

• True cysts: These are easily visualised by US as rounded, smooth-walled anechogenic images that produce PR in the tissue surrounding and posterior to the cyst.

Pathological alterations of the thyroid.
(Localised mixed masses).

• __Haemorrhage or abscess__: They have ill-defined contours with alternating echogenic, hypoechogenic and anechogenic images which are given by fibrin septa in haemorrhages and by pus, detritus and serous elements in abscesses.

Pathological alterations of the thyroid.
(Malignant nodules).

Malignant nodules are more frequent in men and may present as solitary nodules of low echogenicity or complexes of irregular contours and infiltrating nodules that produce distortion of the neighbouring pattern, metastatic adenopathy may be present.

Neck vessels
(carotid and vertebral).

Indications for carotid US.

1   In asymptomatic patients:

-With cervical murmur.

-    With evidence of extracardiac atherosclerosis.
-    With vascular risk factors.

2   In symptomatic patients:

-    With vertigo, loss of consciousness.
-    With amaurosis fugax.
-    With ATI (specify the emboligenic focus).
-    With suspected vertebrobasilar insufficiency.
-    With suspicion of subclavian robbery.
-    In patients with ischaemic heart disease.

3   In control:

-    Pre-surgical patients.
-    Post-surgical patients.
-    Follow-up of patients without surgical criteria.

Preparation.

No prior preparation is required.

The study is performed with the patient in the supine decubitus position, placing a pillow on the head and cervical region or using a bed with dorsal elevation. If possible, a hyperextension of the neck should be achieved to allow the study of the vessels; it is advisable to give a discreet oblique position in the opposite direction to the vessel being explored.

Technique for the study of the vessels of the neck.

Colour and spectral Doppler mode.

- It allows to demonstrate:

-    Permeability of the vessel.
-    Direction of flow.
-    Functional categorisation (haemodynamic significance of the injury assessed).

Colour Doppler ultrasound of the vertebral artery.

-    Normal diameter (4 mm).
-    Variable size.
-    Difficult to visualise
-    Low resistance flows

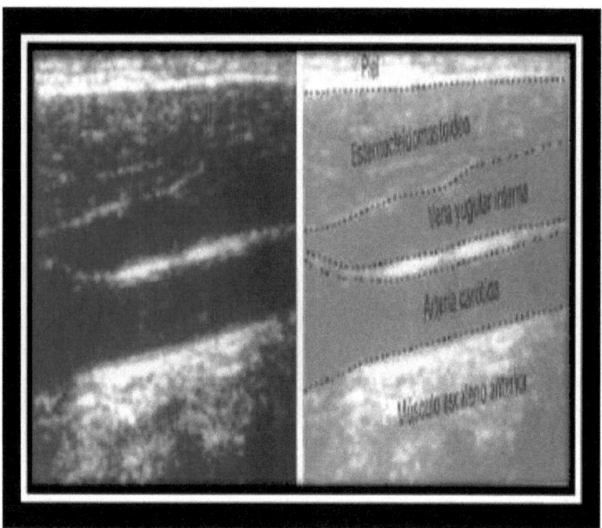

Corte longitudinal de la arteria carótida común y vena yugular interna

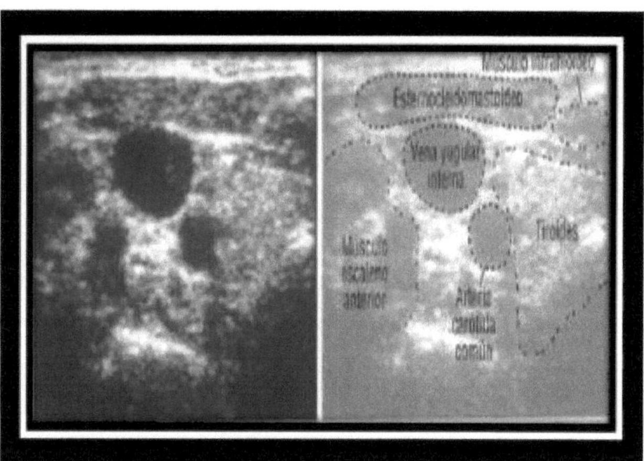

Imagen transversal de carótida común

Cross-section of the normal thyroid gland
Longitudinal section of the thyroid gland with small cystic masses.

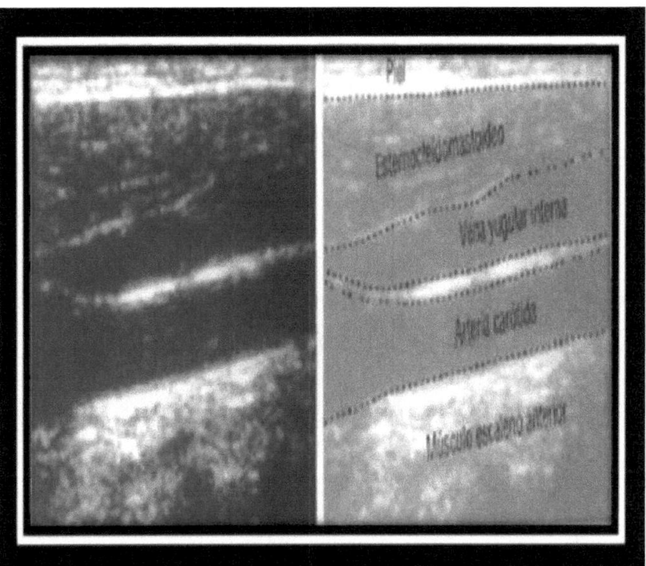

Longitudinal section of the common carotid artery and internal jugular vein.

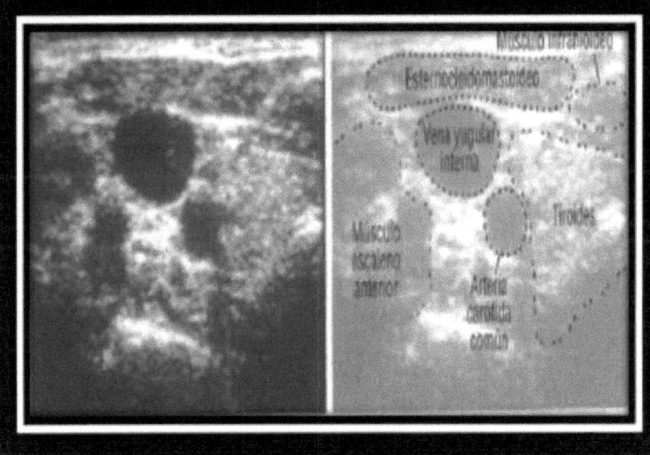

Transverse image of common carotid artery

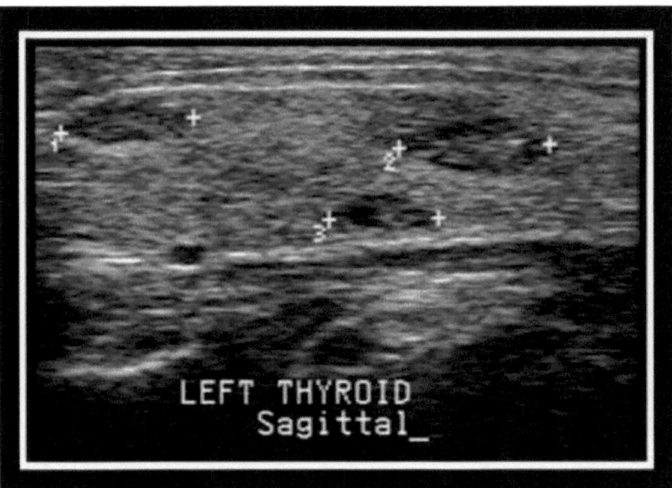

Longitudinal image of the left lobe of the thyroid gland with a multinodular appearance.

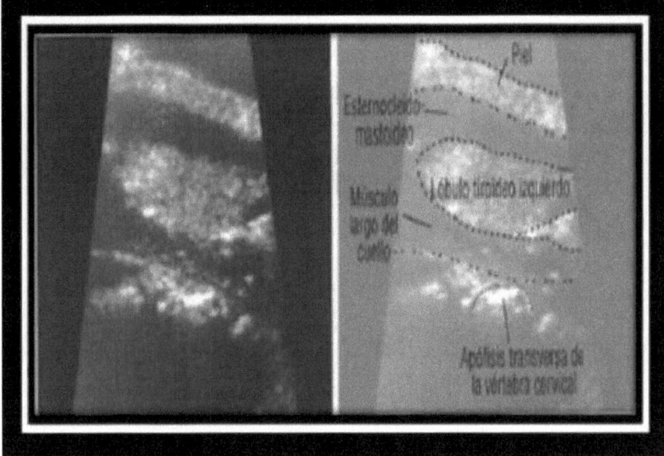

Longitudinal image of the thyroid gland

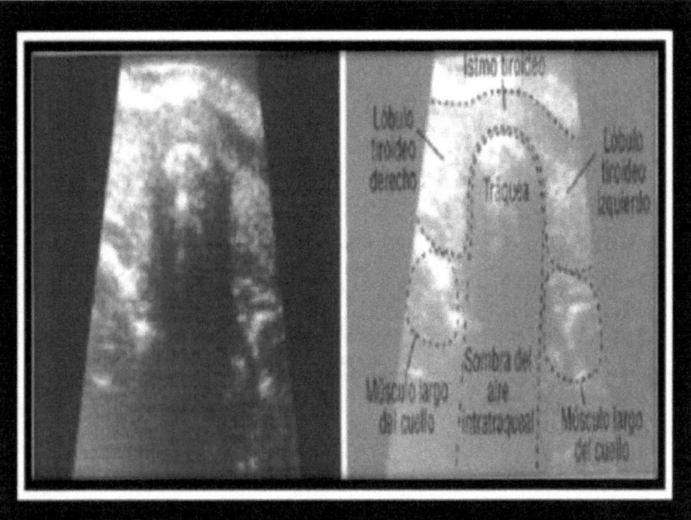

Cross-sectional image of the thyroid gland

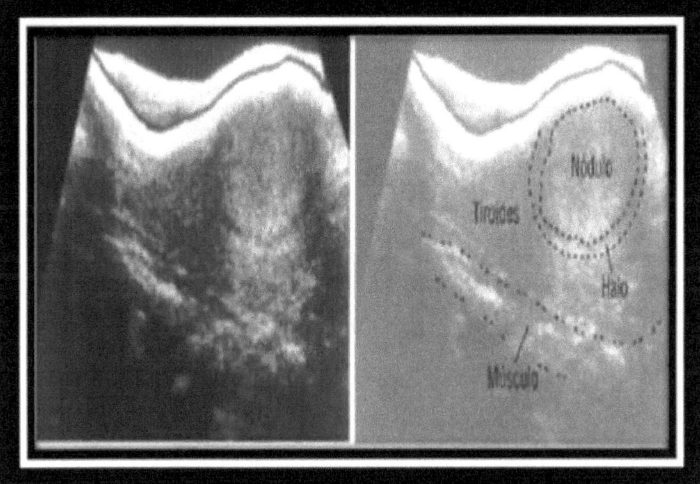

Longitudinal image of isoechoic nodule

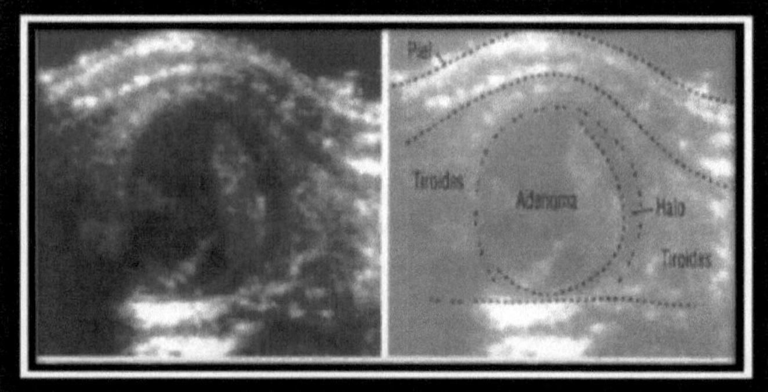

Longitudinal imaging of adenomas and cysts

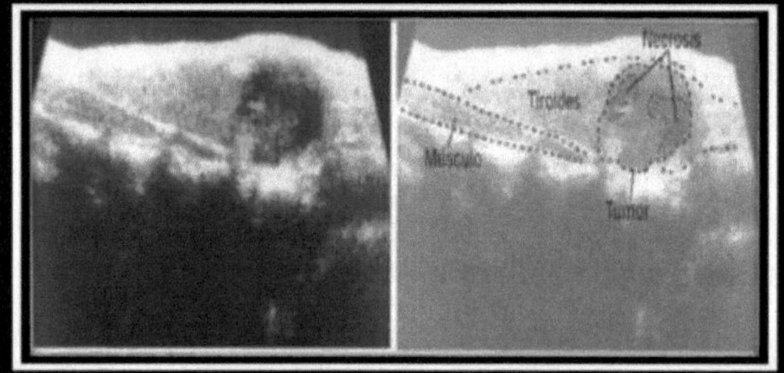

Longitudinal image of carcinoma

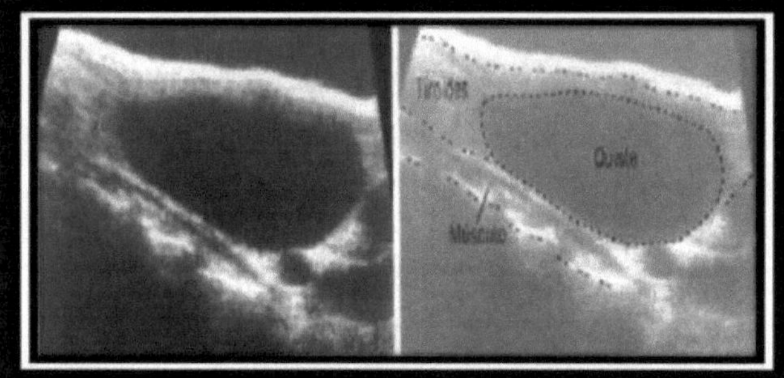

Longitudinal image (thyroid cyst)

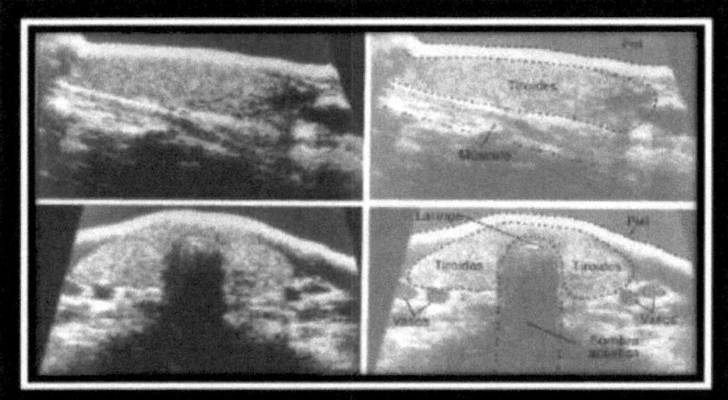

Longitudinal imaging of homogeneous thyroid hyperplasia

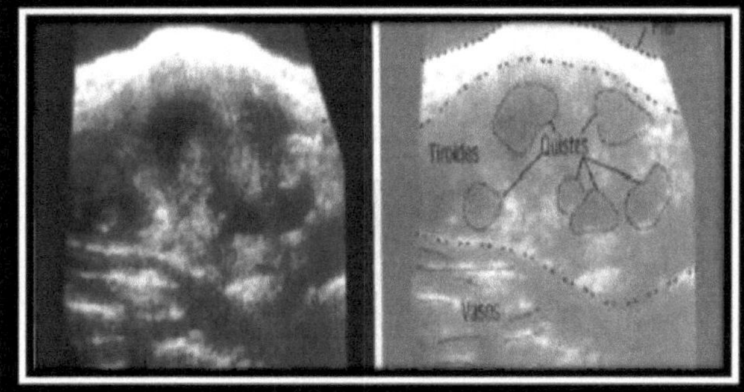

Enlarged heterogeneous thyroid with nodules

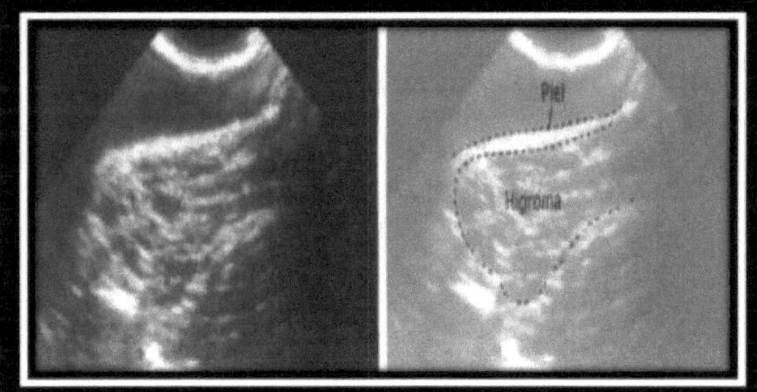

Cystic hygroma

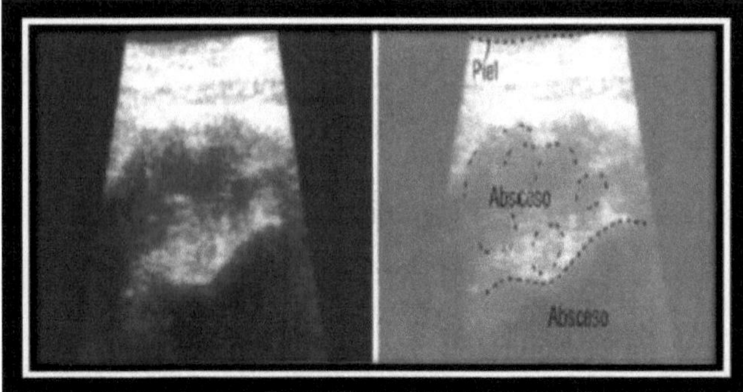

Longitudinal image of retropharyngeal abscess

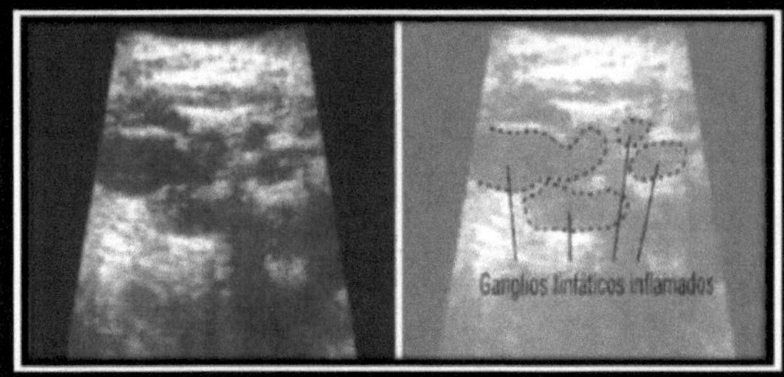

Swollen lymph nodes

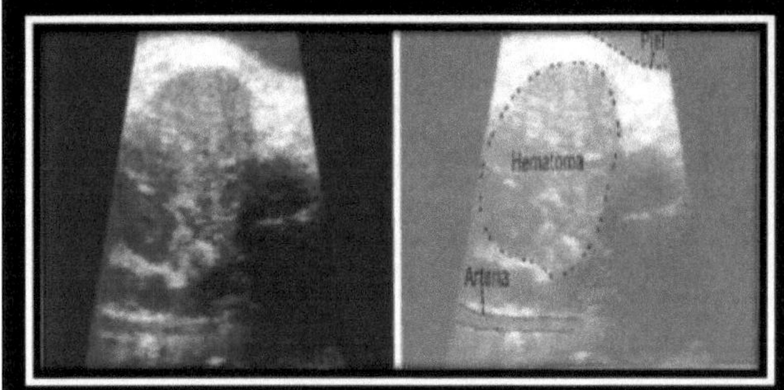

Haematoma

Chapter 16

USD DE MAMA.

Sonographic assessment of breast lesions has become increasingly valuable in recent years, given the adverse reactions women receive from radiation during mammography.

In pregnant women and young women it is the ideal method for the study of breast pathology, while in adult women (patients over 40 years of age) it can be complemented by radiological examinations, especially when a malignant lesion is suspected.

INDICATIONS.

> To assess the nature of a papillary nodular lesion, differentiate between solid, cystic and complex masses.

> To sometimes identify a benign or malignant lesion.

> To periodically evaluate the breasts or for medical check-up.

> For pain or inflammation of the breasts.

NORMAL ANATOMY.

> The breast has a glandular parenchyma containing 15 to 20 lobules, each with small lobules. The mammary gland contains the areola and the nipple into which the milk ducts lead.

> For its study it is divided into 4 quadrants, 2 upper (external and internal) and 2 lower (external and internal) and on the areola we draw the hands of a clock, which allows us to locate the time or place where the lesion is located.

EXAMINATION TECHNIQUE.

Patient in decubitus supine position, checking the 4 quadrants with simultaneous palpation of the breast presided over by the transducer and always directed towards the nipple. If the breast is very small or the lesion is very superficial, we use a bag of water to obtain a better image.

NORMAL SONOGRAPHIC APPEARANCE

> Occasionally the galactophore ducts are observed, in the form of tubular echolucent structures of at least 2 mm in diameter that converge towards the nipple.

PATHOLOGICAL SONOGRAPHIC ASPECTS.

> Cystic or echolucent lesions do not show internal echoes, have well-defined borders, with posterior wall enhancement.

> Solid or echodense lesions and complex lesions show different degrees of echogenicity with posterior sound attenuation.

> Benign nodules have smooth, well-defined borders, while malignant nodules usually have irregular, ill-defined borders.

> There are some breast cancers (non-infiltrating carcinomas) that behave like benign lesions.

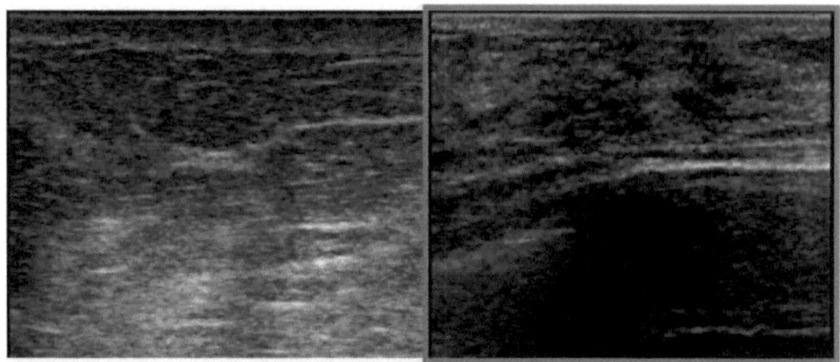

Normal patterns

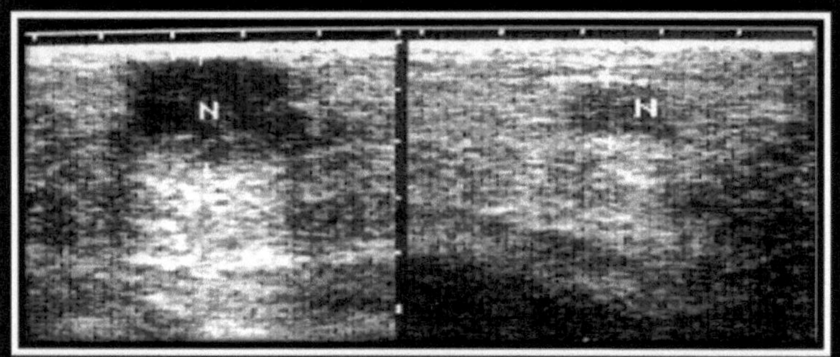

Breast lumps

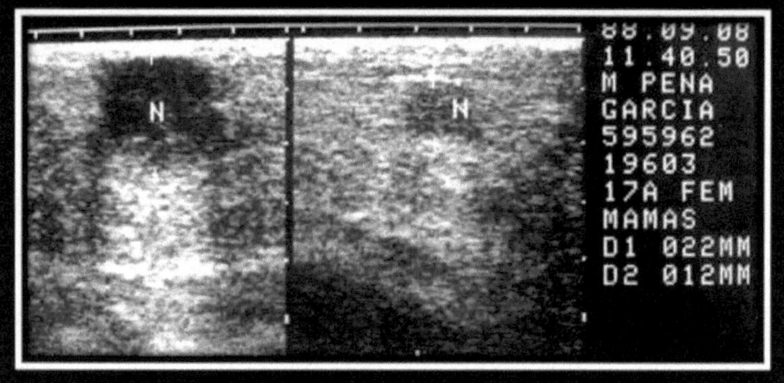

Breast lumps

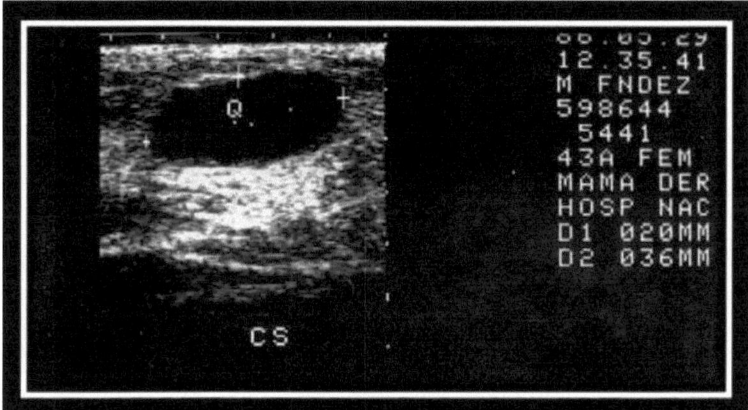

Breast cyst

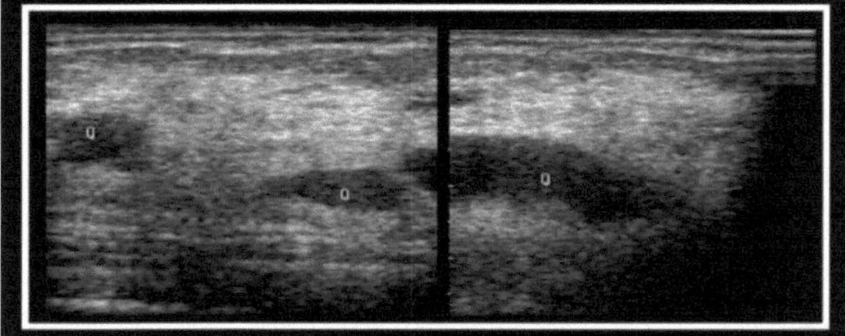

Fibrocystic fibrocystic disease

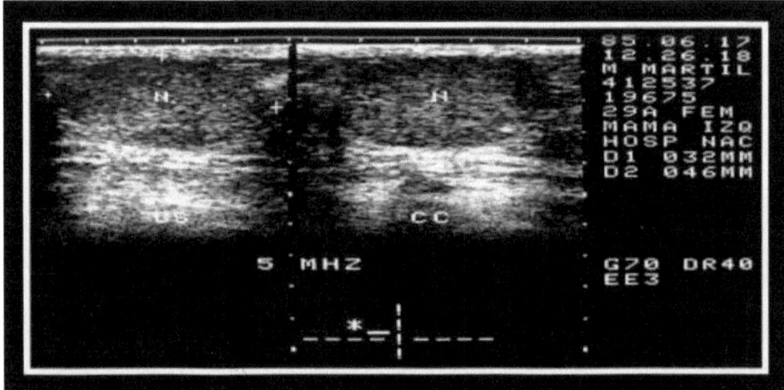

Fibroadenoma

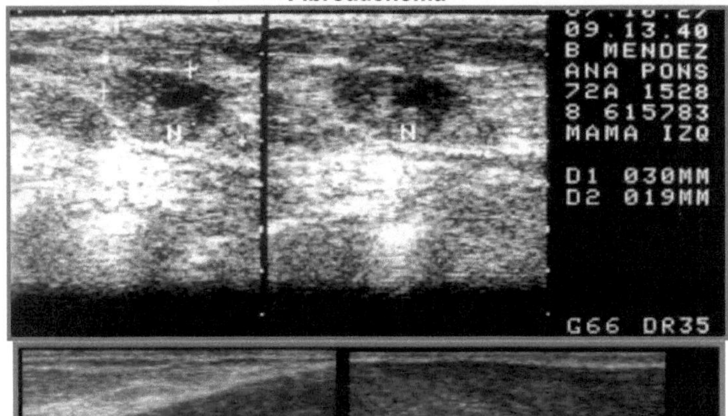

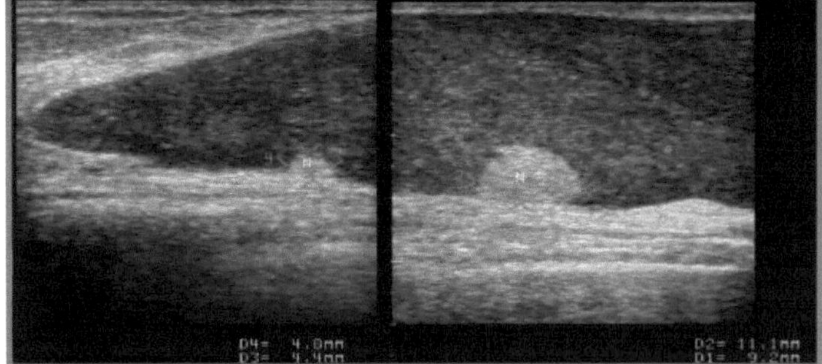

Breast cancer

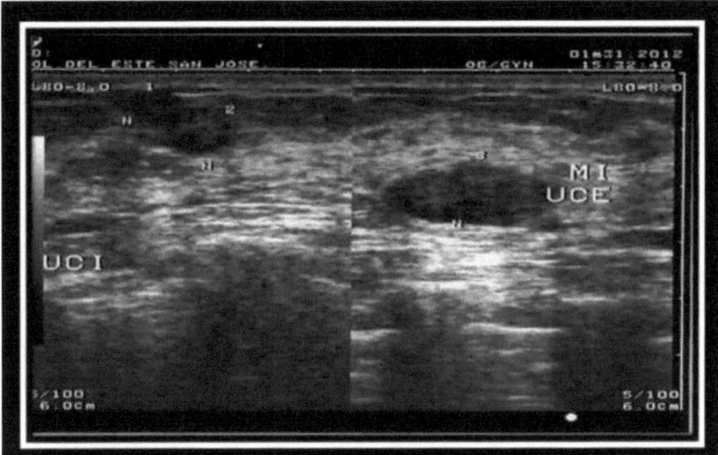

Breast lumps

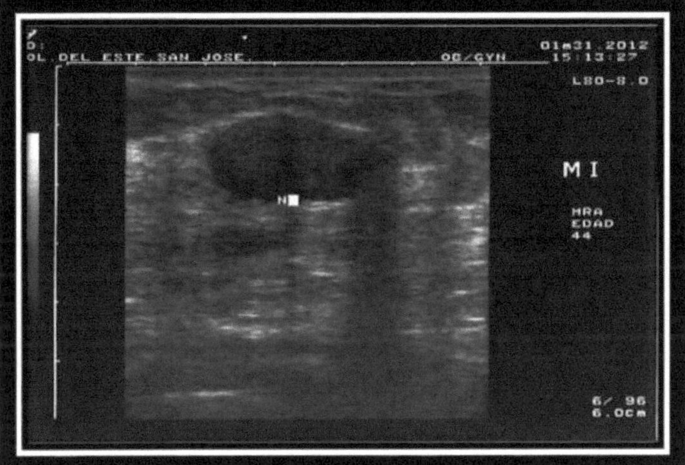

Breast lumps

Bibliograffa

• Abscess of Skene's gland in a newborn. Centro Provincial de Information de Ciencias Medicas de Mayabeque. ISSN 2520-9078 RNPS 2441 RNSW A1269. (2019)

• Acosta Prieto, S. Ultrasonographic diagnosis of acute cholecystitis. Revista Medica Eletronica de Ciego de Avila. Editorial Ciencias Medicas. ISSN 1029-3035 RNPS 1821 RNSW A1235 (2019)

• A-Thrush Ultrasound-vascular-as-why-and-when-dvd-rom. 3rd ed © 2010, 320 pages.

• Baez Pupo, Francisco. D^az Brito, Yoimy. Baez Pupo, Maria M. Ultrasonographic diagnosis of gynaecological pelvic masses. Rev Cubana Obstet Ginecol vol.42 no.2 Ciudad de la Habana Apr.-Jun. 2016

• Birdwell, R.L. Chronic Radiology Series: Top 100 Breast Diagnostics. © 2005, 340 pages.

• Bruguera Carlos A. Abdominal Ecogratia. SALVAT EDITORES, S.A. Mallorca, 41=Barcelona. Spain. 1982

• Charles-Burke; Robert-Dixon High-performance-radiology-interventional-procedures © 2011, 568 pages.

• Clinicas-radiologicas-de-norteamerica-2005-volumen-43-n-3-fundamentos-del-diagnostico-por-imagen-del-torax authors/C-Chiles © 2006, 184 pages.

• Delgado M. Julio C. Apuntes de Crinica Medica, para la Licenciatura en Tecnologia de la Salud. (Digital). FATESA. 20

• D^az Pi, Oscar. Berty Gutierrez, Hedgar. Martinez Morales, Miguel L. Rodriguez Varela, Reynaldo. Alvarez Arias, Arian. Emergency ultrasound performed by surgeons in patients admitted to the Emergency Department. Revista Cubana de Cirug^a, *print version* ISSN 0034-7493version *On-line* ISSN 1561-2945

• Jane-bates. Ultrasound-abdominal-as-why-and-when. 3rd ed © 2011, 360 pages.

• Jamie-Weir; Peter-H-Abrahams; Jonathan-D-Spratt;Lonie-R-Salkowski.atlas-of-human-anatom^a-by-tëimaging-techniques

• Sopena, R; Vilar, J; Marti-Bonmati, L; Algorithms in diagnostic imaging. 2nd ed © 2005, 256 pag.

• Muraoka S, Tsuchida K, Iwasaki M, Izawa N, Jinnai H, Komatsubara T, et al. A case report of gas-tric lymphitis plastica diagnosed by endoscopic ultrasound-guided fine needle aspiration. Medicine (Baltimore) [Internet]. 2017 [cited 4 Sep 2018];96(50):[approx. 5 p.]. Available from: https://www.ncbi.nlm.nih.gov/pmc/articles/PMC5815695/pdf/medi-96-e8937.pdf.

• Nicolas-Sans-Franck-Lapegue Ultrasonography-musculoskeletal. 2011, 320 pages.

• N-Dalrymple.solution-of-problems-in-abdominal-imaging-CD-Rom © 2010, 696 pages.

• Liu YM, Yang XJ. Endoscopic ultrasound-guided cutting of holes and deep biopsy for diagnosis of gastric infiltrative tumors and gastrointestinal submucosal tumors using a novel vertical diathermic loop. World J Gastroenterol [Internet]. 2017 [cited 4 Sep 2018]; 23 (15): [approx. 7p .]. Available in: https://www.ncbi.nlm.nih.gov/pmc/articles/PMC5403759/.

• Llanio N. Reimundo and co-authors. Propedeutica clinica y semiolog^a medica. Volume I. Editorial Ciencias Medicas, 2004.

• Llanio N. Reimundo and co-authors. Propedeutica clmica y semiolog^a medica. Volume II. Editorial Ciencias Medicas, 2004.

• Doors H. Nelson. Gynaeco-obstetric Ultrasound. Editorial Ciencias Medicas. Ciudad de la Habana 2006.

• Kobayashi M. Atlas de Ultrasonograffa en Obstetricia y Ginecolog^a. Editorial Medica Panamericana S.A. VIAMONTE 2164. Buenos Aires.1980.

• Iglesias R. MB. Detection of congenital defects by ultrasound during prenatal diagnosis. Cuban Journal of Medical Genetics. Cuba. Editorial de Ciencias Medicas. ISSN 2070-8718 RNPS 2146. (2018)

• Rose-de-bruyn. Paediatric ultrasound-as-why-and-when. 2nd ed © 2011, 408 pages.

• Roca Goderich, Temas de Medicina Interna. Volume I. Editorial Ciencias Medicas, 5th edition. 2006

• Roca Goderich, Temas de Medicina Interna. Volume II. Editorial Ciencias Medicas, 5th edition. 2006

• Roca Goderich, Temas de Medicina Interna. Volume III. Editorial Ciencias Medicas, 5th edition. 2006

• Rosell Puig, W, Dovale Borjas, C.; Alvarez Torres, I. Morfolog^a Humana I y II. Ciencias Medicas (2002).

• Rosell Puig, W, Dovale Borjas, C.; Alvarez Torres, II. Morfolog^a Humana I y II. Ciencias Medicas (2002).

• Valls Perez Orlando, Hernandez Castro, Jorge Luis and Anillo Bad^a Ricardo. Ecograffa del Aparato locomotor. Editorial Ciencias Medicas, Cuba, 2005.

• Valls. O and Parrilla M. Atlas de Ultrasonido Diagnostico. Editorial Cientffico Tecnica. 1982.

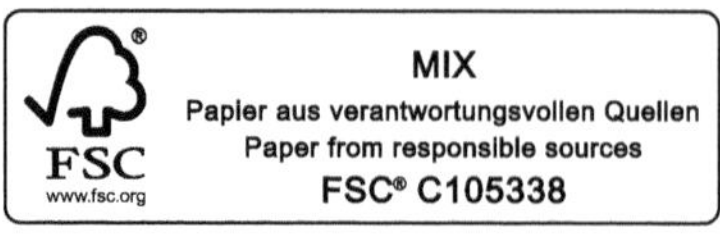

Printed by Books on Demand GmbH, Norderstedt / Germany